Managing Stress: An Evidence Based Guide

Harness the power of proven methods to conquer stress and foster resilience.

Cameron Dunk

Evidence Based Stress Management ©

Managing Stress: An Evidence Based Guide
© 2025 Evidence Based Stress Management
All rights reserved.

Published by:
Evidence Based Stress Management
First published: April 17, 2025
ISBN: 978-1-7642369-0-4

For more information, visit: **www.ebsm.com.au**

Foreword

In today's fast-paced world, stress has become an almost ubiquitous part of daily life, affecting individuals across all walks of life. While numerous stress management techniques are available, not all are grounded in scientific research. This book, "Managing Stress: An Evidence Based Guide," aims to bridge the gap between popular stress relief methods and those that are rigorously supported by empirical evidence.

Drawing from a wealth of scientific studies and clinical trials, this book explores a variety of proven strategies for managing stress effectively. From mindfulness and cognitive-behavioural approaches to physical exercise and nutritional interventions, the book covers a comprehensive range of techniques designed to reduce stress and improve overall well-being.

Readers will gain insights into the physiological and psychological mechanisms of stress, learn how to implement evidence-based strategies in their daily lives, and discover practical tips for maintaining long-term stress resilience. Whether you are a healthcare professional, a student, or simply someone looking to improve your quality of life, this book provides a reliable guide to managing stress through evidence supported methods.

Contents

Introduction

Stress is an inevitable part of life, affecting individuals across all walks of life. It is a natural response to challenging or threatening situations, but when it becomes chronic, it can have detrimental effects on both physical and mental health. While there are many proclaimed stress management methods, not all are supported by research. This book hopes to sift through these various methods and highlight those that are evidence based.

While these methods are thorough and effective, they are not an exhaustive list. It is crucial to consult a medical professional before undertaking any new stress management techniques, especially if you are experiencing significant stress. A healthcare provider can offer personalized advice and ensure that the methods you choose are safe and appropriate for your specific circumstances.

What is Stress?

Stress is a multifaceted concept that encompasses physical, mental, and emotional responses to external pressures. It is a natural part of life, but its effects can vary widely depending on the individual and the context.

Physiological Definition

Stress is often defined as the body's response to any demand or challenge that disrupts its physiological equilibrium. This response involves the activation of the hypothalamus–pituitary-adrenal (HPA) axis, leading to the release of stress hormones such as cortisol and adrenaline (Shahsavarani, Marz Abadi, & Kalkhoran, 2015). These hormones prepare the body for a "fight or flight" response by increasing heart rate, blood pressure, and energy supplies.

Psychological Definition

Stress is perceived as a state of mental or emotional strain resulting from adverse or demanding circumstances (Manosso, Gasparini, Réus, & Pavlovic, 2022). This can include feelings of anxiety, frustration, and overwhelm. Psychological stress is influenced by an individual's perception of their ability to cope with the stressor.

Historical Perspectives

The concept of stress has evolved over time. Hans Selye, often referred to as the "father of stress research", defined stress as the non-specific response of the body to any demand for change (Nater, 2021). Today, stress is recognized as a complex interaction between environmental demands and an individual's ability to cope with those demands. This interaction is influenced by various factors, including genetics, personality, and social support (Nater, 2021). Examples include:

- **Workplace Stress**: Deadlines, workload, and interpersonal conflicts can all contribute to stress at work.
- **Academic Stress**: Students often experience stress due to exams, assignments, and the pressure to perform well.
- **Financial Stress**: Concerns about money and financial stability are common sources of stress.
- **Health-Related Stress**: Chronic illnesses or health concerns can be significant stressors.

Chapter 1

Understanding Stress

Understanding stress is crucial in stress management because it allows us to identify the triggers and physiological responses that contribute to our stress levels. By comprehending the underlying mechanisms of stress, we can better recognize its impact on our health and well-being. This knowledge empowers us to implement effective strategies to mitigate stress, improve our coping mechanisms, and enhance our overall quality of life.

Physiology of Stress – The Autonomic Nervous System (ANS)

The autonomic nervous system (ANS) is a critical component of the nervous system that regulates involuntary physiological functions. It operates largely below the level of consciousness and controls functions such as heart rate, digestion, respiratory rate, pupillary response, urination, and sexual arousal. Understanding the ANS's structure and function is essential in learning how stress can affect the body.

The ANS is divided into three main branches:

1. **Sympathetic Nervous System (SNS):**
   a. **Function:** Often referred to as the "fight or flight" system, the SNS prepares the body to respond to perceived threats. It increases heart rate, dilates airways, and mobilizes energy stores (Kandel, Schwartz, Jessell, Siegelbaum, & Hudspeth, 2013).
   b. **Anatomy:** The SNS originates in the thoracic and lumbar regions of the spinal cord. It uses a two-neuron pathway: preganglionic neurons (short) and postganglionic neurons (long) that communicate in or near the target organs (Kandel, Schwartz, Jessell, Siegelbaum, & Hudspeth, 2013).

2. **Parasympathetic Nervous System (PNS):**
   a. **Function:** Known as the "rest and digest" system, the PNS promotes relaxation and recovery. It decreases heart rate, stimulates digestive processes, and conserves energy (Kandel, Schwartz, Jessell, Siegelbaum, & Hudspeth, 2013).
   b. **Anatomy:** The PNS originates in the brainstem and sacral spinal cord. It also uses a two-neuron pathway: preganglionic neurons (long) and postganglionic

neurons (short) that communicate in or near the target organs (Kandel, Schwartz, Jessell, Siegelbaum, & Hudspeth, 2013).

3. **Enteric Nervous System (ENS):**

   a. **Function:** Often called the "second brain," the ENS controls gastrointestinal functions independently of the Central Nervous System (CNS). It regulates muscle contraction, enzyme secretion, and blood flow within the gut (Bankenahally & Krovvidi, 2016).

   b. **Anatomy:** The ENS consists of a network of neurons embedded in the walls of the gastrointestinal tract (Bankenahally & Krovvidi, 2016).

The ANS operates through a series of reflex arcs that involve sensory (afferent) and motor (efferent) pathways:

- **Afferent Pathways:** These pathways transmit sensory information from the body to the CNS. Receptors in the viscera (e.g. baroreceptors in the aortic arch) detect changes in internal conditions and send signals via cranial nerves (e.g. vagus nerve) to the brainstem (Kandel, Schwartz, Jessell, Siegelbaum, & Hudspeth, 2013).

- **Efferent Pathways:** These pathways carry motor commands from the CNS to the target organs. The efferent limb is divided into preganglionic and postganglionic neurons, which communicate in in or near the target organs (Kandel, Schwartz, Jessell, Siegelbaum, & Hudspeth, 2013).

Examples of ANS Functions

1. **Cardiovascular Regulation:**
   a. **Sympathetic Activation:** Increases heart rate and contractility, constricts blood vessels to raise blood pressure.
   b. **Parasympathetic Activation:** Decreases heart rate and promotes vasodilation (the widening of blood vessels due to the relaxation of the blood vessel's muscular walls) to lower blood pressure.

2. **Digestive System Control:**
   a. **Sympathetic Activation:** Inhibits digestive activities, reduces blood flow to the gastrointestinal tract.
   b. **Parasympathetic Activation:** Stimulates digestive processes, increases blood flow to the gastrointestinal tract.

3. **Respiratory Regulation:**
   a. **Sympathetic Activation:** Dilates bronchioles to increase airflow.
   b. **Parasympathetic Activation:** Constricts bronchioles to decrease airflow.

Hormonal Response: The Role of Cortisol

Cortisol, often referred to as the "stress hormone," plays a crucial role in the body's response to stress. It is produced by the adrenal glands and is involved in a wide range of physiological processes. Understanding cortisol's role and its effects on the body is crucial for developing strategies to manage stress and mitigate its negative health impacts.

Production and Regulation of Cortisol

Cortisol is produced in the adrenal cortex, the outer layer of the adrenal glands, which are located on top of the kidneys. The production and release of cortisol are regulated by the hypothalamic-pituitary-adrenal (HPA) axis:

1. **Hypothalamus:** In response to stress, the hypothalamus releases corticotropin-releasing hormone (CRH).
2. **Pituitary Gland:** CRH stimulates the anterior pituitary gland to secrete adrenocorticotropic hormone (ACTH).
3. **Adrenal Glands:** ACTH travels through the bloodstream to the adrenal glands, prompting them to release cortisol into the bloodstream (James, Stromin, Steenkamp, & Combrinck, 2023).

Functions of Cortisol

1. **Metabolism Regulation:**
   a. **Glucose Metabolism:** Cortisol increases blood sugar levels by promoting gluconeogenesis (the production

of glucose from non-carbohydrate sources) in the liver. This provides immediate energy to respond to stress (Lee, Meyer, Nenke, Lightman, & Torpy, 2024).

b. **Protein and Fat Metabolism:** Cortisol facilitates the breakdown of proteins and fats to provide additional energy sources (Lee, Meyer, Nenke, Lightman, & Torpy, 2024).

2. **Immune Response:**

a. **Anti-Inflammatory Effects:** Cortisol suppresses the immune system's inflammatory response, reducing inflammation and preventing overreaction to stress (Sapolsky, Romero, & Munck, 2000).

b. **Immunosuppression:** While beneficial in the short term, prolonged cortisol exposure can weaken the immune system, making the body more susceptible to infections (Sapolsky, Romero, & Munck, 2000).

3. **Cardiovascular Function:**

a. **Blood Pressure Regulation:** Cortisol helps maintain blood pressure by increasing the sensitivity of blood vessels to catecholamines (e.g. adrenaline). This ensures adequate blood flow during stress (Ullian, 1999).

4. **Central Nervous System:**
   a. **Mood and Cognition:** Cortisol influences mood, motivation, and fear responses. It affects areas of the brain involved in memory and learning, such as the hippocampus (Law & Clow, 2020).

Types of Stress

Acute Stress: Short-Term Stress and its Immediate Effects
Acute stress is a type of stress that occurs in response to an immediate perceived threat or challenge. It is short-term and typically resolves once the stressor is removed. While acute stress can be beneficial in certain situations by enhancing performance and focus, it can also have immediate physiological and psychological effects. Understanding the mechanisms and effects of acute stress can help you develop strategies to manage stress effectively and harness its potential benefits.

When faced with an acute stressor, the body undergoes a series of rapid physiological changes, often referred to as the "fight or flight" response. This response is primarily mediated by the sympathetic nervous system (SNS) and the hypothalamic-pituitary-adrenal (HPA) axis (Ernst et al., 2023).

Physiological responses to acute stress include:

1. **Activation of the Sympathetic Nervous System (SNS):**
   a. **Heart Rate and Blood Pressure:** The SNS increases heart rate and blood pressure to ensure that more oxygen and nutrients are delivered to vital organs and muscles (Ernst et al., 2023).
   b. **Respiratory Rate:** Breathing rate increases to supply more oxygen to the bloodstream (Ernst et al., 2023).
   c. **Energy Mobilization:** The body releases glucose and fatty acids into the bloodstream to provide immediate energy (Ernst et al., 2023).

2. **Hypothalamic-Pituitary-Adrenal (HPA) Axis Activation:**
   a. **Cortisol Release:** The HPA axis stimulates the release of cortisol from the adrenal glands. Cortisol helps maintain energy supply by increasing blood sugar levels and enhancing the metabolism of fats, proteins, and carbohydrates (Weber, Angerer, & Apolinário-Hagen, 2022).
   b. **Adrenaline and Noradrenaline:** These hormones are released to prepare the body for rapid action. They increase heart rate, blood pressure, and energy availability (Weber, Angerer, & Apolinário-Hagen, 2022).

Immediate effects of acute stress include:

1. **Enhanced Cognitive Function:**
   a. **Increased Alertness:** Acute stress can improve alertness and concentration, helping individuals respond quickly to the stressor (Shahsavarani, Marz Abadi, & Kalkhoran, 2015).
   b. **Memory Formation:** Short-term stress can enhance memory formation, making it easier to remember important details related to the stressor (Shahsavarani, Marz Abadi, & Kalkhoran, 2015).

2. **Physical Reactions:**
   a. **Muscle Tension:** Muscles may become tense as the body prepares for potential physical action (Shahsavarani, Marz Abadi, & Kalkhoran, 2015).
   b. **Sweating:** Increased sweating helps cool the body during heightened physical activity (Shahsavarani, Marz Abadi, & Kalkhoran, 2015).

3. **Emotional Responses:**
   a. **Anxiety and Fear:** Acute stress often triggers feelings of anxiety and fear, which can motivate individuals to take action to avoid or confront the stressor (Shahsavarani, Marz Abadi, & Kalkhoran, 2015).

b. **Irritability:** Some individuals may experience irritability or frustration in response to acute stress (Shahsavarani, Marz Abadi, & Kalkhoran, 2015).

Examples of acute stress in everyday life include:

- **Public Speaking:** The anticipation of giving a speech can trigger acute stress, leading to increased heart rate, sweating, and heightened alertness.
- **Exams:** Students often experience acute stress before and during exams, which can enhance focus and memory recall.
- **Emergency Situations:** Encountering a sudden emergency, such as a car accident, can induce acute stress, prompting quick decision-making and physical responses.

Episodic Acute Stress: Frequent Acute Stress Episodes and Their Impact

Episodic acute stress refers to frequent episodes of acute stress, often resulting from a lifestyle filled with chaos, high demands, and constant pressure. Unlike acute stress, episodic acute stress occurs in spurts but can still have significant health implications if not managed properly. Individuals experiencing episodic acute stress often live in a state of constant tension and anxiety. Understanding the mechanisms and effects of episodic acute stress can help you develop strategies to manage stress effectively and mitigate its negative health impacts.

Physiological responses to episodic acute stress include:

1. **Sympathetic Nervous System (SNS) Activation:**
   a. **Heart Rate and Blood Pressure:** Frequent activation of the SNS leads to repeated increases in heart rate and blood pressure, which can strain the cardiovascular system over time (Ernst et al., 2023).
   b. **Energy Mobilization:** Each episode of acute stress mobilizes energy by releasing glucose and fatty acids into the bloodstream, which can disrupt metabolic processes if it occurs too often (Ernst et al., 2023).

2. **Hypothalamic-Pituitary-Adrenal (HPA) Axis Activation:**
   a. **Cortisol Release:** Episodic acute stress triggers the release of cortisol, which helps the body manage the immediate stressor. However, frequent spikes in cortisol can lead to dysregulation of the HPA axis (Weber, Angerer, & Apolinário-Hagen, 2022).
   b. **Adrenaline and Noradrenaline:** These hormones are released during each stress episode, preparing the body for rapid action but also contributing to wear and tear on the body (Weber, Angerer, & Apolinário-Hagen, 2022).

Immediate and long-term effects of episodic acute stress include:

1. **Cardiovascular Health:**
   a. **Hypertension:** Repeated episodes of acute stress can lead to sustained high blood pressure, increasing the risk of hypertension and cardiovascular diseases (Khan & Khan, 2017).
   b. **Heart Disease:** Frequent stress responses can cause inflammation and damage to the arteries, contributing to the development of heart disease (Khan & Khan, 2017).

2. **Mental Health:**
   a. **Anxiety and Panic Attacks:** Individuals with episodic acute stress are more likely to experience anxiety and panic attacks due to the constant activation of the stress response (Halbreich, 2021).
   b. **Depression:** The persistent feeling of being overwhelmed can lead to depressive symptoms over time (Halbreich, 2021).

3. **Cognitive Function:**
   a. **Memory Impairment:** Frequent stress episodes can impair memory and cognitive function, particularly affecting the hippocampus, which is involved in

memory formation (Woo, Hong, Jung, Choe, & Yu, 2018).

b. **Attention Deficits:** Episodic acute stress can reduce the ability to concentrate and focus, impacting productivity and daily functioning (Sherman, Huang, Wijaya, Turk-Browne, & Goldfarb, 2024)

Examples of Episodic acute stress in everyday life include:

- **High-Pressure Jobs:** Professionals in high-stress occupations, such as emergency responders, surgeons, and stock traders, often experience episodic acute stress due to the nature of their work.

- **Multitasking and Overcommitment:** Individuals who juggle multiple responsibilities, such as working parents or students with heavy course loads, may frequently encounter acute stress episodes.

- **Perfectionism and Pessimism:** People with perfectionist tendencies or a pessimistic outlook may experience episodic acute stress as they constantly worry about meeting high standards or anticipate negative outcomes.

Chronic Stress: Long-Term Stress and its Detrimental Effects on Health

Chronic stress is a prolonged and persistent state of stress that can have significant negative impacts on both physical and mental health. It exerts continuous pressure on the body and mind, leading to various health issues including cardiovascular disease, depression, and weakened immune function (Halbreich, 2021). By understanding the wide-ranging impacts of chronic stress, you can better address and manage this pervasive issue, improving overall health and quality of life.

The physiological impacts of chronic stress include:

1. **Cardiovascular System:**
    a. **Hypertension:** Chronic stress can lead to sustained high blood pressure, increasing the risk of heart disease and stroke. The continuous release of stress hormones like cortisol and adrenaline causes blood vessels to constrict, raising blood pressure (Khan & Khan, 2017).
    b. **Heart Disease:** Prolonged stress is associated with an increased risk of developing coronary artery disease. Stress hormones can cause inflammation and damage to the arteries, contributing to plaque buildup and heart attacks (Khan & Khan, 2017).
2. **Immune System:**
    a. **Immunosuppression:** Chronic stress suppresses the immune system, making the body more susceptible to infections and illnesses. This is due to the prolonged release of cortisol, which inhibits the production of

cytokines necessary for immune response (Halbreich, 2021).

b. **Inflammation:** Persistent stress can lead to chronic inflammation, which is linked to various diseases, including autoimmune disorders and cancer. Stress-induced inflammation is a result of the immune system's overreaction to prolonged stress (Halbreich, 2021).

3. **Gastrointestinal System:**

a. **Digestive Issues:** Stress can affect the digestive system, leading to conditions such as irritable bowel syndrome (IBS) and exacerbating symptoms of gastrointestinal disorders. Stress alters gut motility and increases sensitivity to pain in the digestive tract (Shchaslyvyi, Antonenko, & Telegeev, 2024).

b. **Appetite Changes:** Chronic stress can cause changes in appetite, leading to weight gain or loss. Stress can trigger emotional eating or loss of appetite, affecting nutritional intake and overall health (Shchaslyvyi, Antonenko, & Telegeev, 2024).

The neurological impacts of chronic stress include:

1. **Brain Structure and Function:**

a. **Hippocampus:** Chronic stress can reduce the volume of the hippocampus, a brain region critical for learning and memory. This can impair memory consolidation and increase the risk of neurodegenerative diseases like Alzheimer's (Blum, 2024).

b. **Amygdala:** The amygdala, which regulates emotions and threat detection, becomes hyperactive under chronic stress. This can lead to heightened anxiety, fear responses, and emotional instability (Zhang et al., 2018).

c. **Prefrontal Cortex:** Prolonged stress can cause atrophy in the prefrontal cortex, affecting executive functions such as decision-making, impulse control, and cognitive flexibility (Datta & Arnsten, 2019).

2. **Neurochemical Changes:**

a. **Cortisol Dysregulation:** Chronic stress leads to dysregulation of cortisol. Elevated cortisol levels can impair cognitive function and increase the risk of mental health disorders (Knezevic, Nenic, Milanovic, & Knezevic, 2023).

b. **Neurotransmitter Imbalances:** Stress affects the balance of neurotransmitters like serotonin and dopamine, which are crucial for mood regulation. Imbalances in these chemicals can lead to depression and anxiety (Sharma, 2024).

The psychological impacts of chronic stress include:

1. **Mental Health Disorders:**

   a. **Depression:** Chronic stress is a significant risk factor for depression. It can lead to persistent feelings of sadness, hopelessness, and a lack of interest in activities (Lei et al., 2025).

   b. **Anxiety Disorders:** Prolonged stress can cause or exacerbate anxiety disorders, characterized by excessive worry, fear, and panic attacks (Mah, Claudia, & Alexandra, 2016).

   c. **Post-Traumatic Stress Disorder (PTSD):** Individuals exposed to chronic stress, especially traumatic events, are at higher risk of developing PTSD. Symptoms include flashbacks, severe anxiety, and uncontrollable thoughts about the event (Miao, Chen, Wei, Tao, & Lu, 2018).

2. **Cognitive Impairments:**

   a. **Memory Problems:** Chronic stress can impair both short-term and long-term memory. The hippocampus, which is involved in memory formation, is particularly vulnerable to stress-induced damage (Krugers, Lucassen, Karst, & Joëls, 2010).

b. **Attention Deficits:** Stress can reduce the ability to concentrate and focus, affecting productivity and daily functioning (Halkos & Bousinakis, 2010).

Examples of chronic stress in everyday life include:

- **Work-Related Stress:** High job demands, lack of control, and job insecurity can contribute to chronic stress. Long hours, tight deadlines, and workplace conflicts are common stressors.
- **Financial Stress:** Ongoing financial difficulties, such as debt and unemployment, are common sources of chronic stress. Financial insecurity can lead to constant worry and anxiety.
- **Chronic Illness:** Living with a long-term health condition can be a significant source of stress. Managing symptoms, treatment regimens, and the emotional toll of illness contribute to chronic stress.

As we transition from understanding the multifaceted nature of stress and its profound effects on both the mind and body, it becomes imperative to explore the various techniques that have been researched and shown to manage and mitigate these impacts. The remainder of this book delves into a range of stress management strategies, each backed by studies and expert recommendations. From ancient practices like yoga and meditation to modern interventions such as nutrition and Cognitive-Behavioural Therapy (CBT), these techniques offer practical solutions to help navigate the complexities of stress in our daily lives. By integrating these methods, you can not only alleviate the immediate symptoms of stress but also foster long-term resilience and well-being.

Chapter 2

Lifestyle Modifications and Stress Management

We will now look at lifestyle modifications for stress management. It is important to consider these as they can significantly improve your overall well-being, enhance your ability to cope with stress, and prevent the negative health effects associated with chronic stress. By making thoughtful changes to your daily habits and routines, you can build resilience, improve mental clarity, and foster a healthier, more balanced life.

Importance of Quality of Sleep: How Sleep Affects Stress Levels and Overall Health

Quality sleep is essential for maintaining overall health and well-being. It plays a crucial role in regulating stress levels, supporting cognitive function, and promoting physical health. Poor sleep quality can exacerbate stress and lead to a range of health issues. Understanding the importance of quality sleep and its impact on stress levels and overall health can help you prioritize sleep and adopt healthy sleep habits to improve your well-being.

How Sleep Affects Stress Levels

1. **Regulation of Stress Hormones:**

   a. **Cortisol Levels:** Quality sleep helps regulate cortisol, the primary stress hormone. During sleep, cortisol levels naturally decrease, allowing the body to recover from daily stress. Poor sleep can disrupt this cycle, leading to elevated cortisol levels and increased stress (Lo Martire, Berteotti, Zoccoli, & Bastianini, 2024).

   b. **Sympathetic Nervous System (SNS) Activity:** Adequate sleep reduces the activity of the sympathetic nervous system, which is responsible for the "fight or flight" response. This helps lower stress and anxiety levels (Lo Martire, Berteotti, Zoccoli, & Bastianini, 2024).

Impact of Sleep on Overall Health

1. **Cognitive Function:**

   a. **Memory Consolidation:** Sleep plays a critical role in memory consolidation. During sleep, the brain processes and stores information from the day, enhancing learning and memory. Poor sleep can impair cognitive function and memory (Blaxton, Bergeman, Whitehead, Braun, & Payne, 2017).

   b. **Attention and Concentration:** Quality sleep improves attention, concentration, and problem-solving skills. Sleep deprivation can lead to difficulties in focusing and making decisions (Blaxton, Bergeman, Whitehead, Braun, & Payne, 2017).

2. **Physical Health:**

   a. **Immune System Function:** Sleep is vital for a healthy immune system. It enhances the body's ability to fight infections and reduces inflammation. Chronic sleep deprivation can weaken the immune system, making individuals more susceptible to illnesses (Garbarino, Lanteri, Bragazzi, Magnavita, & Scoditti, 2021).

   b. **Metabolic Health:** Quality sleep helps regulate metabolism and maintain a healthy weight. Poor sleep is associated with an increased risk of obesity, diabetes, and metabolic syndrome (Kim et al., 2018).

3. **Cardiovascular Health:**

   a. **Blood Pressure Regulation:** Sleep helps regulate blood pressure by reducing sympathetic nervous system activity. Poor sleep can lead to hypertension and increase the risk of cardiovascular diseases (Khan & Khan, 2017).

   b. **Heart Health:** Adequate sleep is essential for heart health. It reduces the risk of heart disease by lowering blood pressure, reducing inflammation, and improving overall cardiovascular function (Khan & Khan, 2017).

Improving sleep quality involves various practices that promote restful and uninterrupted sleep. These include establishing a regular sleep schedule, creating a restful environment, and avoiding stimulants before bedtime. By adopting these sleep hygiene practices, you can improve your sleep quality, reduce stress levels, and enhance overall health and well-being.

1) **Establishing a Regular Sleep Schedule**

Maintaining a consistent sleep schedule is crucial for regulating the body's internal clock, also known as the circadian rhythm. This helps improve the quality and duration of sleep.

- **Consistency**: Go to bed and wake up at the same time every day, even on weekends. This consistency reinforces your body's sleep-wake cycle.
- **Sleep Duration**: Aim for 7-9 hours of sleep per night, as recommended by sleep experts (Watson et al., 2015). Adequate sleep duration is associated with better health outcomes, including reduced risk of chronic diseases (Flinders University, 2024).
- **Bedtime Routine**: Develop a relaxing pre-sleep routine to signal to your body that it's time to wind down. This

could include activities such as reading, taking a warm bath, or practicing relaxation exercises.

2) Creating a Restful Environment

The sleep environment plays a significant role in determining sleep quality. A conducive sleep environment minimizes disruptions and promotes relaxation.

- **Noise Reduction:** Minimize noise in the bedroom. Use earplugs, white noise machines, or heavy curtains to block out disruptive sounds (Czeisler, Buxton, & Dzierzewski, 2023).

- **Light Control:** Keep the bedroom dark by using blackout curtains or an eye mask. Exposure to light, especially blue light from screens, can interfere with the production of melatonin, a hormone that regulates sleep (Czeisler, Buxton, & Dzierzewski, 2023).

- **Comfortable Bedding:** Invest in a comfortable mattress and pillows that support your preferred sleeping position. The right bedding can significantly enhance sleep quality (Czeisler, Buxton, & Dzierzewski, 2023).

- **Temperature:** Maintain a cool room temperature, ideally between 15-19°C (60-67°F). A cooler environment helps facilitate the body's natural drop in temperature during sleep (Czeisler, Buxton, & Dzierzewski, 2023).

The following sleep aids have been found to help in providing a restful sleep environment for individuals and improve their quality of sleep:

- **Red Light Therapy (RLT)**: has been studied for its potential benefits in managing stress through various physiological and psychological mechanisms. RLT works by penetrating the skin and stimulating cellular function, which can reduce oxidative stress and inflammation (Hamblin, 2017). Additionally, RLT has been shown to positively affect mood and anxiety levels (Pan, Zhang, Deng, Lin, & Pan, 2023). Furthermore, RLT can improve sleep quality by promoting melatonin production, as RLT can improve sleep onset and overall sleep quality (Pan, Zhang, Deng, Lin, & Pan, 2023).

- **Sleep Masks**: Sleep masks, often used to block out light and improve sleep quality, have been studied for their potential benefits in stress management. Sleep masks work by blocking out ambient light, which can help improve sleep quality. It has been found that wearing an eye mask during overnight sleep improved episodic learning and alertness the next day (Greco et al., 2023). Additionally, sleep masks are found to reduce the frequency of night wakings and improve overall sleep quality (Bahcecioglu Turan, Gürcan, & Özer, 2023).

- **Nasal Strips:** Nasal strips, commonly used to alleviate nasal congestion, have been studied for their potential benefits in improving sleep quality and reducing stress. Nasal strips work by mechanically opening the nasal passages, which can improve airflow and reduce nasal congestion. It has been found that nasal strips significantly improved subjective measures of sleep quality in individuals with chronic nasal congestion (Schenkel, Ciesla, & Shanga, 2018).

3) Avoiding Stimulants Before Bedtime

Stimulants can interfere with the ability to fall asleep and stay asleep. It's important to avoid consuming stimulants close to bedtime.

- **Caffeine:** Avoid caffeine-containing beverages and foods at least 6 hours before bedtime. Caffeine is a central nervous system stimulant that can delay sleep onset and reduce sleep quality (Marks, 2020).
- **Nicotine:** Refrain from smoking or using nicotine products before bed. Nicotine is a stimulant that can disrupt sleep patterns and lead to insomnia (Marks, 2020).
- **Alcohol:** While alcohol may initially induce drowsiness, it can disrupt sleep later in the night and reduce overall

sleep quality. It's best to avoid alcohol close to bedtime (Marks, 2020).

An alternative can be drinking peppermint tea before bed. Research suggests that peppermint may alleviate stress through its calming aroma and muscle-relaxing properties (Abdelhalim, 2021). The key compound in peppermint, menthol, has been shown to have a soothing effect on the nervous system, which can help reduce stress levels (Abdelhalim, 2021).

Exercise and Stress Reduction: The Benefits of Regular Physical Activity in Mitigating Stress

Regular physical activity is one of the most effective ways to manage and reduce stress. Exercise has numerous physiological and psychological benefits that contribute to overall well-being and resilience against stress. Understanding these benefits can help you incorporate regular physical activity into your routines to manage stress and improve overall health.

Physiological Benefits of Exercise

1. **Reduction of Stress Hormones:**
   a. **Cortisol Levels:** Exercise helps lower cortisol levels (Torres, Koutakis, & Forsse, 2021). Regular physical activity promotes the release of endorphins, which

counteract the effects of cortisol and induce feelings of well-being.

b. **Adrenaline and Noradrenaline**: Physical activity helps regulate the release of adrenaline and noradrenaline, reducing the body's overall stress response (Heijnen, Hommel, Kibele, & Colzato, 2016).

2. **Improved Cardiovascular Health**:

a. **Heart Rate and Blood Pressure**: Regular exercise strengthens the cardiovascular system, leading to lower resting heart rate and blood pressure. This reduces the strain on the heart and blood vessels during stressful situations (Pinckard, Baskin, & Stanford, 2019).

b. **Enhanced Blood Flow**: Exercise improves circulation, ensuring that oxygen and nutrients are efficiently delivered to tissues and organs, which helps the body recover from stress more effectively (Pinckard, Baskin, & Stanford, 2019).

3. **Enhanced Immune Function**:

a. **Immune System Boost**: Moderate exercise enhances immune function by promoting the circulation of immune cells, which helps the body fight off infections and reduces inflammation (Romeo, Wärnberg, Pozo, & Marcos, 2010).

b. **Reduced Inflammation:** Regular physical activity helps lower chronic inflammation, which is often exacerbated by stress (Pahomov, Kostunina, & Artemenkov, 2024).

Psychological Benefits of Exercise

1. **Mood Enhancement:**

    a. **Endorphin Release:** Exercise stimulates the release of endorphins, also known as "feel-good" hormones. These chemicals act as natural painkillers and mood elevators, reducing feelings of stress and anxiety (Singh et al., 2023).

    b. **Serotonin and Dopamine:** Physical activity increases the levels of serotonin and dopamine, neurotransmitters that play a key role in mood regulation and overall mental health (Marques et al., 2021).

2. **Improved Sleep Quality:**

    a. **Sleep Regulation:** Regular exercise helps regulate sleep patterns by promoting deeper and more restful sleep. Improved sleep quality, in turn, reduces stress levels and enhances overall well-being (Korkutata, Korkutata, & Lazarus, 2024).

b. **Reduced Insomnia:** Exercise can alleviate symptoms of insomnia, making it easier to fall asleep and stay asleep (Korkutata, Korkutata, & Lazarus, 2024).

3. **Cognitive Function and Mental Clarity:**

a. **Enhanced Cognitive Function:** Physical activity improves cognitive function, including memory, attention, and problem-solving skills. This helps individuals manage stress more effectively by enhancing their ability to think clearly and make decisions (Singh et al., 2025).

b. **Neurogenesis:** Exercise promotes the growth of new neurons in the brain, particularly in the hippocampus, which is involved in learning and memory (Liu & Nusslock, 2018).

Aerobic Exercises and Stress Reduction

Aerobic exercises, also known as cardiovascular or endurance exercises, involve continuous and rhythmic physical activity that increases heart rate and breathing. Examples include running, cycling, swimming, and dancing.

1. **Benefits for Stress Management:**

a. **Reduction of Stress Hormones:** Aerobic exercise helps lower levels of cortisol and adrenaline, the body's primary stress hormones. It also stimulates the production of endorphins, which are natural mood elevators and painkillers (Singh et al., 2023).

b. **Improved Cardiovascular Health:** Regular aerobic exercise strengthens the heart and improves circulation, which can help mitigate the physical effects of stress on the body (Pinckard, Baskin, & Stanford, 2019).

c. **Enhanced Mood and Mental Health:** Aerobic exercise has been shown to reduce symptoms of anxiety and depression. It promotes the release of neurotransmitters like serotonin and dopamine, which play a key role in mood regulation (Marques et al., 2021).

Strength Training and Stress Reduction

Strength training, also known as resistance training, involves exercises that improve muscle strength and endurance. This can include weightlifting, bodyweight exercises, and resistance band workouts.

1. **Benefits for Stress Management:**
   a. **Reduction of Anxiety and Depression:** Strength training has been shown to reduce symptoms of anxiety and depression. It helps regulate neurotransmitters and promotes a sense of accomplishment and control

(Prochilo, Costa, Hassed, Chambers, & Molenberghs, 2021).

b. **Improved Self-Esteem and Confidence**: Regular strength training can enhance self-esteem and body image, which can reduce stress and improve overall mental health (Prochilo, Costa, Hassed, Chambers, & Molenberghs, 2021).

c. **Enhanced Cognitive Function**: Strength training has been linked to improved cognitive function, including better memory and attention. This can help individuals manage stress more effectively by enhancing their ability to think clearly and make decisions (Singh et al., 2025).

Yoga and Pilates: Their Effectiveness in Managing Stress

Yoga and Pilates are both widely recognized for their potential to manage stress through various physiological and psychological mechanisms. Yoga has been shown to reduce stress by regulating the autonomic nervous system and the hypothalamic-pituitary-adrenal (HPA) axis, enhancing interoceptive awareness, which improves emotional regulation and reduces stress (Pascoe et al., 2017). It has been found that mindfulness-based interventions, including yoga, are effective in reducing stress, anxiety, and depression (Hofmann & Gómez, 2017).

Similarly, Pilates promotes physical relaxation and improves body awareness, significantly reducing cortisol levels and improving mood (Byrnes, Wu, & Whillier, 2017). Additionally, Pilates can enhance mental well-being by improving focus and concentration (Caldwell et al., 2009). Overall, evidence supports the effectiveness of both yoga and Pilates in stress management by reducing cortisol levels, improving mood, and enhancing mental clarity.

Balanced Diet: The Impact of Nutrition on Mood and Stress Levels

A balanced diet plays a crucial role in maintaining mental health and managing stress. The nutrients we consume can significantly influence brain function, mood regulation, and overall psychological well-being. We recommend consulting with your doctor or dietician before making any significant changes to your diet.

Key Nutrients and Their Effects on Mood and Stress

1. **Omega-3 Fatty Acids:**
   a. **Function:** Omega-3 fatty acids are essential for brain function and development. They help reduce inflammation and support neurotransmitter function,

which can improve mood and reduce stress (Horovitz, 2025).

    b. **Impact on Mood:** Studies have shown that omega-3 fatty acids can help alleviate symptoms of depression and anxiety by enhancing the production of serotonin, a neurotransmitter that regulates mood (Horovitz, 2025).

Sources: Fatty fish (salmon, mackerel, sardines), flaxseeds, chia seeds, walnuts.

2. **B Vitamins:**

    a. **Function:** B vitamins, including B6, B12, and folate, are crucial for energy production and the synthesis of neurotransmitters (Owen & Corfe, 2017).

    b. **Impact on Mood:** Adequate intake of B vitamins supports cognitive function and emotional stability. Deficiencies in these vitamins have been linked to increased risk of depression and mood disorders (Owen & Corfe, 2017).

Sources: Whole grains, legumes, leafy greens, eggs, dairy products.

3. **Magnesium:**

    a. **Function:** Magnesium is involved in over 300 biochemical reactions in the body, including muscle and nerve function, and the regulation of blood pressure. It aids in muscle relaxation and can help alleviate physical symptoms of stress, such as muscle tension and cramps (Kris-Etherton et al., 2021).

b. **Impact on Stress:** Magnesium has a calming effect on the nervous system and can help reduce symptoms of anxiety and stress (Kris-Etherton et al., 2021).

Sources: Leafy greens (spinach, kale), nuts (almonds, cashews), seeds (pumpkin seeds, sunflower seeds), whole grains.

4. **Vitamin D:**

a. **Function:** Vitamin D is crucial for bone health, immune function, and mood regulation.

b. **Impact on Mood:** Low levels of vitamin D have been associated with increased risk of depression (Anglin, Samaan, Walter, & McDonald, 2013).

Sources: Sunlight exposure, fatty fish (salmon, mackerel), fortified dairy products, egg yolks.

5. **Antioxidants:**

a. **Function:** Antioxidants, such as vitamins C and E, protect the body from oxidative stress and inflammation (Chen, Touyz, Park, & Schiffrin, 2001).

b. **Impact on Stress:** A diet rich in antioxidants can help reduce oxidative stress and improve overall mental health (Sharifi-Rad et al., 2020).

Sources: Fruits (berries, citrus fruits), vegetables (broccoli, spinach), nuts, seeds.

6. **Fermented Foods**

   c. **Function:** Fermented foods introduce beneficial bacteria (probiotics) into the gut, promoting a balanced microbiome.

   d. **Impact on Stress:** Probiotics in fermented foods can influence brain chemistry by regulating neurotransmitters and reducing inflammation, which can help reduce anxiety and depression (Yu et al., 2020). This is through reducing activity in the amygdala, a brain region involved in stress and emotions (Yu et al., 2020).

Sources: Yogurt, kimchi, miso, sauerkraut, kefir.

Time Management: Managing your Time Effectively to Reduce Stress

Research supports the effectiveness of time management in stress management through its ability to improve productivity and reduce the physiological effects of stress. By helping you organize your tasks and maintain focus, time management can be a valuable tool in your stress management toolkit.

Physiological Effects of Time Management

Effective time management can reduce stress by helping you feel more in control of your tasks and responsibilities. For example, it has been found that nursing students who practiced effective time management experienced lower levels of stress compared to those who did not (Eldeeb & Eldosoky, 2016). This suggests that time management tools and strategies can help reduce the physiological effects of stress by promoting better organization and task completion.

Impact on Productivity and Stress Levels

Time management strategies, such as the Pomodoro Technique, can improve productivity and reduce stress by breaking work into manageable intervals. The Pomodoro Technique, which involves working for 25 minutes followed by a 5-minute break, can help maintain focus and prevent burnout. Time management strategies help individuals focus on results and identify activities that contribute to efficiency, thereby reducing stress (Singh, 2017).

Emotional and Psychological Benefits

Effective time management can also improve emotional regulation and increase self-awareness. For example, it has been found that students who used time management techniques reported lower levels of anxiety and higher levels of academic performance (Eissa & Kader, 2015). This indicates that time management can help you better understand and manage your emotions, leading to reduced stress.

Examples of Time Management Techniques

- **Pomodoro Technique:** Work for 25 minutes, then take a 5-minute break. After four cycles, take a longer break of 15-30 minutes.
- **Time Blocking:** Allocate specific blocks of time for different tasks throughout the day to ensure all responsibilities are addressed.
- **Prioritization:** Identify and focus on high-priority tasks to ensure that the most important work is completed first.

Chapter 3

Relaxation Techniques

We will now look at relaxation techniques for stress management. It is important to consider these techniques because they can significantly reduce the physical and mental effects of stress, promoting overall well-being. These practices also enhance mental clarity, improve mood, and increase resilience to stress. By incorporating relaxation techniques into your daily routine, you can better manage stress and improve your quality of life

Progressive Muscle Relaxation (PMR): Technique Overview

Progressive Muscle Relaxation (PMR) is a technique designed to reduce physical tension and stress by systematically tensing and then relaxing different muscle groups in the body. This method can help you become more aware of the physical sensations associated with tension and relaxation, promoting overall relaxation and stress reduction (Gangadharan & Madani, 2018).

Concept and Mechanism

a. **Tension and Relaxation:** PMR involves deliberately tensing specific muscle groups for a few seconds and then releasing the tension. This process helps distinguish between the sensations of tension and relaxation, making it easier to identify and reduce muscle tension in daily life (Kumutha, Aruna, & Poongodi, 2014).

b. **Autonomic Nervous System:** By promoting relaxation, PMR activates the parasympathetic nervous system, which counteracts the "fight or flight" response of the sympathetic nervous system. This leads to a decrease in heart rate, blood pressure, and overall stress levels (Kumutha, Aruna, & Poongodi, 2014).

Step-by-Step Guide to PMR

1. **Find a Comfortable Space:**

   a. **Preparation:** Choose a quiet, comfortable place where you won't be disturbed. You can sit or lie down in a relaxed position. A quiet room with dim lighting and a comfortable chair or bed is ideal for practicing PMR.

2. **Take Deep Breaths:**

   a. **Relaxation:** Close your eyes and take a few deep breaths. Inhale slowly through your nose, hold for a few seconds, and exhale slowly through your mouth. This helps calm your mind and prepare your body for relaxation. Inhale for a count of four, hold for a count of four, and exhale for a count of six.

3. **Start with Your Feet:**

   a. **Tensing:** Begin with your feet. Curl your toes tightly and hold the tension for about 5-10 seconds.

   b. **Releasing:** Gradually release the tension and focus on the sensation of relaxation for about 15-20 seconds. Notice the difference between the tension in your toes and the relaxation that follows.

4. **Progress Upwards:**

   a. **Calves:** Point your toes upward, flexing your calves. Hold the tension for 5-10 seconds, then release and relax.

   b. **Thighs:** Squeeze your thigh muscles tightly. Hold for 5-10 seconds, then release and relax.

   c. **Abdomen:** Tighten your abdominal muscles as if preparing for a punch. Hold for 5-10 seconds, then release and relax.

   d. **Chest:** Take a deep breath and hold it, expanding your chest. Hold for 5-10 seconds, then exhale and relax.

   e. **Hands:** Clench your fists tightly. Hold for 5-10 seconds, then release and relax.

   f. **Arms:** Bend your elbows and tense your biceps. Hold for 5-10 seconds, then release and relax.

g. **Shoulders:** Shrug your shoulders up toward your ears. Hold for 5-10 seconds, then release and relax.

h. **Neck:** Press your head back gently, tensing the neck muscles. Hold for 5-10 seconds, then release and relax.

i. **Face:** Scrunch your facial muscles, including your forehead, eyes, and mouth. Hold for 5-10 seconds, then release and relax.

5. **Visualization and Affirmations (Optional):**

a. **Visualization:** As you relax each muscle group, visualize the tension melting away. Imagine a wave of relaxation flowing through your body.

b. **Affirmations:** Use positive affirmations to enhance relaxation. For example, silently repeat, "I am calm and relaxed" as you release tension.

6. **Enjoy Complete Relaxation:**

a. **Final Relaxation:** After you've worked through all the muscle groups, take a few moments to enjoy the overall sense of relaxation. Focus on your breathing and the feeling of calmness. Spend 2-3 minutes in this state of complete relaxation, allowing your body and mind to fully unwind.

1. **Physical Relaxation:** PMR helps reduce muscle tension, which is often a physical manifestation of stress. By systematically relaxing muscles, you can alleviate physical discomfort and promote overall relaxation (Gangadharan & Madani, 2018).

2. **Mental Calmness:** The focus required for PMR can divert attention from stressors, promoting mental calmness and reducing anxiety (Gangadharan & Madani, 2018).

3. **Improved Sleep:** Regular practice of PMR can improve sleep quality by reducing physical and mental tension before bedtime (Gangadharan & Madani, 2018).

4. **Enhanced Awareness:** PMR increases body awareness, helping you recognize early signs of stress and tension, allowing for timely intervention (Gangadharan & Madani, 2018).

Diaphragmatic Breathing: Techniques for Deep Breathing to Activate the Body's Relaxation Response

Diaphragmatic breathing, also known as deep breathing or abdominal breathing, is a technique that involves engaging the diaphragm to achieve full oxygen exchange and promote relaxation. This method can help activate the body's relaxation response, reducing stress and improving overall well-being. By incorporating diaphragmatic breathing into daily routines, you can effectively manage stress and enhance your overall quality of life.

Mechanism and Physiology

a. **Diaphragm Function:** The diaphragm is a large, dome-shaped muscle located at the base of the lungs. When you breathe in deeply, the diaphragm contracts and moves downward, allowing the lungs to expand and fill with air. When you exhale, the diaphragm relaxes and moves upward, helping to expel air from the lungs (Hamasaki, 2020).

b. **Autonomic Nervous System:** Diaphragmatic breathing stimulates the parasympathetic nervous system, which counteracts the "fight or flight" response of the sympathetic nervous system. This leads to a decrease in heart rate, blood pressure, and overall stress levels (Hamasaki, 2020).

Step-by-Step Guide to Practicing Diaphragmatic Breathing

1. **Find a Comfortable Position:**
   a. **Preparation:** Sit or lie down in a comfortable position. Place one hand on your chest and the other on your abdomen to feel the movement of your diaphragm.

2. **Inhale Deeply:**
   a. **Technique:** Inhale slowly through your nose, allowing your abdomen to rise as your diaphragm contracts. Your chest should remain relatively still. Imagine filling your abdomen with air like a balloon. Count to four as you inhale.

3. **Hold the Breath:**
   a. **Technique:** Hold your breath for a few seconds to allow for maximum oxygen exchange.

4. **Exhale Slowly·**
   a. **Technique:** Exhale slowly through your mouth, allowing your abdomen to fall as your diaphragm relaxes. Your chest should remain relatively still. Imagine slowly deflating the balloon. Count to six as you exhale.

5. **Repeat the Process:**

    a. **Technique:** Continue this pattern of deep breathing for several minutes, focusing on the rise and fall of your abdomen. Aim for 5-10 minutes of diaphragmatic breathing, gradually increasing the duration as you become more comfortable with the technique.

Examples of Diaphragmatic Breathing Exercises

1. **4-7-8 Breathing:**

    a. **Inhale:** Inhale deeply through your nose for a count of four.

    b. **Hold:** Hold your breath for a count of seven.

    c. **Exhale:** Exhale slowly through your mouth for a count of eight.

2. **Box Breathing:**

    a. **Inhale:** Inhale deeply through your nose for a count of four.

    b. **Hold:** Hold your breath for a count of four.

    c. **Exhale:** Exhale slowly through your mouth for a count of four.

    d. **Hold:** Hold your breath for a count of four before starting the next inhale.

Benefits of Diaphragmatic and Deep Breathing

Physiological benefits include:

1. **Activation of the Parasympathetic Nervous System:**

a. **Mechanism:** Deep breathing stimulates the parasympathetic nervous system (PNS), which is responsible for the "rest and digest" response. This activation helps counterbalance the "fight or flight" response triggered by the sympathetic nervous system (SNS) during stress (Perciavalle et al., 2017).

b. **Impact:** By promoting parasympathetic activity, deep breathing reduces heart rate, lowers blood pressure, and decreases levels of stress hormones like cortisol and adrenaline (Perciavalle et al., 2017).

2. **Improved Oxygenation:**

a. **Mechanism:** Deep breathing enhances oxygen exchange in the lungs, increasing oxygen delivery to tissues and organs. This improved oxygenation supports overall cellular function and energy production (Bentley et al., 2023).

b. **Impact:** Better oxygenation helps reduce physical symptoms of stress, such as muscle tension and fatigue, and promotes a sense of well-being (Bentley et al., 2023).

3. **Reduction of Muscle Tension:**

a. **Mechanism:** Deep breathing encourages relaxation of the diaphragm and other respiratory muscles, which can help release tension in the body (Jerath, Crawford, Barnes, & Harden, 2015).

b. **Impact:** Reduced muscle tension alleviates physical discomfort and promotes a state of relaxation, making it easier to manage stress and anxiety (Jerath, Crawford, Barnes, & Harden, 2015).

Psychological benefits include:

1. **Enhanced Emotional Regulation:**

   a. **Mechanism:** Deep breathing helps regulate emotions by promoting mindfulness and present-moment awareness. This practice can reduce the intensity of negative emotions and enhance emotional stability (Perciavalle et al., 2017).

   b. **Impact:** Improved emotional regulation helps you respond to stressors more calmly and effectively, reducing overall anxiety levels.

2. **Reduction of Anxiety Symptoms:**

   a. **Mechanism:** Deep breathing techniques have been shown to reduce symptoms of anxiety by lowering physiological arousal and promoting relaxation (Bentley et al., 2023).

   b. **Impact:** Regular practice of deep breathing can lead to significant reductions in anxiety symptoms, improving overall mental health and quality of life.

3. **Improved Cognitive Function:**

   a. **Mechanism:** Deep breathing enhances cognitive function by increasing oxygen delivery to the brain and reducing the impact of stress on cognitive processes (Tsakona et al., 2025).

   b. **Impact:** Better cognitive function helps you think more clearly, make better decisions, and manage stress more effectively.

Mindfulness Meditation: Staying Present and Focused to Reduce Stress

Mindfulness meditation is a practice that involves maintaining a moment-by-moment awareness of thoughts, feelings, bodily sensations, and the surrounding environment. It emphasizes acceptance and non-judgment, allowing you to stay present and focused. By incorporating mindfulness meditation into daily routines, you can effectively manage stress, improve emotional regulation, and enhance your overall quality of life.

Concept and Mechanism

   a. **Present-Centred Awareness:** Mindfulness meditation encourages you to focus on the present moment rather than ruminating on the past or worrying about the future. This present-centred awareness helps reduce stress by breaking the cycle of negative thought patterns (Chems-Maarif, Cavanagh, Baer, Gu, & Strauss, 2025).

b. **Non-Judgmental Attitude**: Practicing mindfulness involves observing thoughts and feelings without judgment. This non-judgmental attitude fosters acceptance and reduces the emotional impact of stressors (Chems-Maarif, Cavanagh, Baer, Gu, & Strauss, 2025).

Step-by-Step Guide to Practicing Mindfulness Meditation

1. **Find a Quiet Space**:
   a. **Preparation**: Choose a quiet, comfortable place where you won't be disturbed. Sit or lie down in a relaxed position. A quiet room with dim lighting and a comfortable cushion or chair is ideal for practicing mindfulness meditation.

2. **Focus on Your Breath**:
   a. **Technique**: Close your eyes and take a few deep breaths. Focus on the sensation of your breath entering and leaving your body. Notice the rise and fall of your abdomen or the feeling of air passing through your nostrils. Inhale deeply through your nose for a count of four, hold for a count of four, and exhale slowly through your mouth for a count of six.

3. **Observe Your Thoughts and Feelings:**
    a. **Technique:** As you continue to breathe deeply, observe any thoughts, feelings, or sensations that arise. Acknowledge them without judgment and gently bring your focus back to your breath. If you notice your mind wandering, simply note the distraction and return your attention to your breath.

4. **Practice Non-Judgmental Awareness:**
    a. **Technique:** Maintain a non-judgmental attitude towards your thoughts and feelings. Accept them as they are without trying to change or suppress them. If you feel anxious, acknowledge the feeling without labelling it as "bad" or "wrong." Simply observe it and let it pass.

5. **Gradually Increase Duration:**
    a. **Technique:** Start with short sessions of 5-10 minutes and gradually increase the duration as you become more comfortable with the practice. Aim to practice mindfulness meditation for 20-30 minutes daily for optimal benefits.

Examples of Mindfulness Meditation Practices

1. **Body Scan Meditation:**
    a. **Technique:** This practice involves mentally scanning your body from head to toe, paying attention to any

sensations, tension, or discomfort. It helps increase body awareness and promote relaxation. Lie down in a comfortable position and slowly bring your attention to each part of your body, starting from your toes and moving up to your head.

2. **Loving-Kindness Meditation:**

   a. **Technique:** This practice involves focusing on feelings of love and compassion towards yourself and others. It helps cultivate positive emotions and reduce negative feelings and reducing levels of cortisol (Reilly & Stuyvenberg, 2023). Sit comfortably and silently repeat phrases such as "May I be happy, may I be healthy, may I be safe," gradually extending these wishes to others.

Benefits of Mindful Meditation

Physiological benefits include:

a. **Activation of the Parasympathetic Nervous System:** Mindfulness meditation activates the parasympathetic nervous system, promoting relaxation and reducing the physiological effects of stress, such as elevated heart rate and blood pressure (Allen, Romate, & Rajkumar, 2021).

b. **Reduction of Stress Hormones:** Regular mindfulness practice can lower levels of cortisol, thereby reducing overall stress levels (Allen, Romate, & Rajkumar, 2021).

Psychological benefits include:

a. **Enhanced Emotional Regulation:** Mindfulness meditation improves emotional regulation by increasing awareness of emotional responses and promoting a balanced perspective (Eberth & Sedlmeier, 2012).

b. **Reduction of Anxiety and Depression:** Studies have shown that mindfulness meditation can significantly reduce symptoms of anxiety and depression by promoting a sense of calm and improving mood (Eberth & Sedlmeier, 2012).

Aromatherapy: The Effectiveness of Essential Oils in Stress Management

Aromatherapy has been studied extensively for its potential to manage stress. Aromatherapy involves the use of essential oils extracted from plants to improve physical and psychological well-being.

Concept and Mechanism

a. **Olfactory System Stimulation:** The primary mechanism through which aromatherapy is believed to work is by stimulating the olfactory system, which then sends signals to the brain's limbic system, an area that influences emotions, behaviour, and memory. This can lead to physiological responses such as reduced heart rate, lower blood pressure, and decreased levels of stress hormones like cortisol (Herz, 2009).

How to Use Essential Oils

Essential oils can be used in various ways for stress management. We recommend consulting with your doctor before using essential oils as they may interact with medications, exacerbate certain health conditions, and cause allergic reactions.

1. **Inhalation:** This is the most common method, where essential oils are diffused into the air using a diffuser.
2. **Topical Application:** Essential oils can be diluted with a carrier oil and applied to the skin. Common areas include the wrists, temples, and the back of the neck.
3. **Baths:** Adding a few drops of essential oil to a warm bath can provide a relaxing experience.
4. **Massage:** Incorporating essential oils into a massage can enhance relaxation and stress relief.

The following essential oils have been found to assist in stress relief:

1. **Lavender Oil:** Known for its calming properties, lavender oil has been shown to significantly increase salivary secretory immunoglobulin A (s-IgA) levels,

indicating reduced stress (Takagi, Nakagawa, Hirata, Ohta, & Shimoeda, 2019).

2. **Bergamot Oil:** Often used for its uplifting and calming effects, bergamot oil is part of essential oil blends that have been studied for their stress-relieving properties (Saiyudthong, Chansiri, Lee, Sittiprapaporn, & Sathirachawan, 2025).

3. **Ylang-Ylang Oil:** This oil is known for its ability to promote relaxation and reduce anxiety, making it a common component in stress-relief blends (Saiyudthong, Chansiri, Lee, Sittiprapaporn, & Sathirachawan, 2025).

Benefits of Essential Oils in Reducing Stress

1. **Reduction in Stress and Anxiety:** Studies have shown that aromatherapy can significantly reduce stress and anxiety levels (Paula, Luís, Pereira, & João, 2017).

2. **Improved Immune Function:** Aromatherapy with lavender have been shown to significantly increase salivary s-IgA levels, indicating enhanced immune function and reduced stress (Takagi, Nakagawa, Hirata, Ohta, & Shimoeda, 2019).

3. **Lowered Cortisol Levels:** Long-term use of essential oil blends has been found to significantly reduce salivary

cortisol levels, a marker of stress (Saiyudthong, Chansiri, Lee, Sittiprapaporn, & Sathirachawan, 2025).

Fidget Tools: Their Effectiveness in Reducing Stress

Fidget tools are designed to help manage stress, anxiety, and improve focus by providing a physical outlet for nervous energy. They are often used by individuals with ADHD, anxiety disorders, or anyone who finds that keeping their hands busy helps them concentrate or relax.

Concept and Mechanism

a. **Sensory-motor self-regulation:** The primary mechanism through which these tools work is by engaging the user's sense of touch and providing a repetitive, soothing motion that can help to calm the mind and body. This process is known as sensory-motor self-regulation, which can help to release neurotransmitters that stimulate attention and reduce cognitive load (Persia, 2023).

How to Use Fidgets and Calming Rings

1. **Fidget Spinners:** Hold the spinner between your thumb and finger and spin it with a flick of your other hand. Focus on the spinning motion and the sensation it creates.

2. **Fidget Cubes:** These cubes have various tactile features like buttons, switches, and dials. Use them by pressing, flipping, or rotating the different components.

3. **Calming Rings:** Wear the ring on your finger and rotate or slide it back and forth. This can be done discreetly in various settings, such as during meetings or while studying.

Benefits of Fidgets Tools in Reducing Stress

1. **Reduced Anxiety:** Fidget tools can help reduce anxiety by providing a physical outlet for nervous energy, which can calm the nervous system and reduce somatic symptoms of anxiety (Persia, 2023).

2. **Improved Focus:** By engaging in repetitive, soothing motions, fidget tools can help improve focus and attention, particularly in individuals with ADHD (Koiler, Schimmel, Bakhshipour, Shewokis, & Getchell, 2022),

3. **Stress Relief:** The tactile engagement provided by fidget tools can help to lower stress levels by promoting relaxation and reducing cognitive load (Persia, 2023).

Hot and Cold Therapy: Its Effectiveness in Body Relaxation and Stress Management

Hot and cold therapy can be effective methods for managing stress. Hot therapy, such as warm baths or saunas, help to relax muscles, improve circulation, and promote a sense of calm. Cold therapy, including ice baths or cold showers, can reduce inflammation and invigorate the body, providing a refreshing and stress-relieving effect. However, it is important to consult your doctor before trying these methods. Consulting a healthcare professional ensures that these therapies are safe for your specific health conditions and that you use them correctly to avoid potential adverse effects.

Cold Therapy - Ice Baths

Ice baths, also known as cold-water immersion (CWI), have been studied for their potential benefits in stress management through various physiological and psychological mechanisms. Ice baths work by exposing the body to cold temperatures, which can reduce inflammation and muscle soreness. Studies are somewhat limited in this area, but we have included the findings thus far below.

Concept and Mechanism

They involve immersing the body in cold water for a set period. The primary mechanism through which ice baths are believed to work is by reducing inflammation and muscle soreness, enhancing recovery, and potentially improving mental health. The cold exposure triggers vasoconstriction, which reduces blood flow to the muscles, thereby decreasing inflammation and swelling. Upon exiting the ice bath, vasodilation occurs, increasing blood flow and aiding in the removal of metabolic waste products (Bleakley & Davison, 2010).

Benefits of Ice Baths in Reducing Stress

1. **Reduced Muscle Soreness:** Ice baths help reduce delayed onset muscle soreness (DOMS) by decreasing inflammation and muscle damage (Hohenauer et al., 2015).

2. **Enhanced Recovery:** Athletes often use ice baths to speed up recovery between training sessions, allowing them to maintain high performance levels (Hohenauer et al., 2015).

3. **Improved Mental Health:** Cold water immersion has been shown to increase levels of endorphins and norepinephrine, which can improve mood and reduce stress (Huttunen, Kokko, & Ylijukuri, 2004).

4. **Increased Resilience to Stress:** Regular exposure to cold water coupled with breathing exercises can decrease stress levels (Kopplin & Rosenthal, 2022).

Hot Therapy – Saunas

Saunas have been used for centuries for their therapeutic benefits, and modern research supports their effectiveness in stress management. Saunas work by exposing the body to high temperatures, which can trigger a range of physiological responses, including the activation of the autonomic nervous system.

Concept and Mechanism

The primary mechanism through which saunas are believed to work is by inducing a state of hyperthermia, which triggers a range of physiological responses. These responses include increased heart rate, improved circulation, and the release of endorphins, which are natural painkillers and mood elevators. Additionally, the heat exposure helps to reduce cortisol levels, thereby promoting relaxation and reducing stress (Huhtaniemi & Laukkanen, 2020).

Benefits of Saunas in Reducing Stress

1. **Reduced Stress and Anxiety:** Saunas help reduce cortisol levels and increase the production of endorphins, leading to lower stress and anxiety (Hussain & Cohen, 2018).

2. **Improved Cardiovascular Health:** Regular sauna use has been linked to a reduced risk of sudden cardiac death, fatal coronary heart disease, and overall mortality (Hussain & Cohen, 2018).

3. **Enhanced Mood and Energy:** The heat exposure and subsequent physiological responses can lead to improved mood and increased energy levels (Hussain & Cohen, 2018).

4. **Better Sleep:** The relaxation effects of saunas can contribute to improved sleep quality (Hussain & Cohen, 2018).

Chapter 4

Cognitive-Behavioural Therapy (CBT)

Principles of Cognitive-Behavioural Therapy (CBT): Managing Stress by Changing Thought Patterns

Cognitive-Behavioural Therapy (CBT) is a widely used psychotherapeutic approach that helps you manage stress by changing maladaptive thought patterns and behaviours. It is based on the cognitive model of mental illness, which posits that our thoughts, emotions, and behaviours are interconnected. By understanding and applying the principles of CBT, you can effectively manage stress, improve emotional regulation, and enhance your overall quality of life.

Consulting a healthcare professional before starting CBT ensures that your therapy is tailored to your specific needs and that you receive proper guidance throughout the process.

Core Principles of CBT

1. **Cognitive Model:**

   a. **Concept:** The cognitive model, initially developed by Aaron Beck, suggests that it is not the situation itself that causes emotional distress, but rather the individual's interpretation of the situation (Fenn &

Byrne, 2013). For example, if someone interprets a challenging situation as a threat, they may experience anxiety. Conversely, if they view it as an opportunity, they may feel motivated.

b. **Application:** CBT helps you identify and challenge distorted or irrational thoughts (cognitive distortions) and replace them with more balanced and realistic ones (Fenn & Byrne, 2013).

2. **Cognitive Restructuring:**

a. **Concept:** Cognitive restructuring involves identifying and challenging negative automatic thoughts and core beliefs that contribute to emotional distress (Nakao, Shirotsuki, & Sugaya, 2021). Core beliefs are deeply held views about oneself, others, and the world, often formed early in life.

b. **Application:** Through techniques such as socratic questioning and thought records, you learn to examine the evidence for and against your negative thoughts and develop more adaptive beliefs (Nakao, Shirotsuki, & Sugaya, 2021).

3. **Behavioural Activation:**

a. **Concept:** Behavioural activation focuses on increasing engagement in positive and meaningful activities to counteract the avoidance and inactivity often associated with depression and anxiety (Baker, Skolnik, Park, Sprich, & Wilhelm, 2023).

b. **Application:** You are encouraged to schedule and participate in activities that bring you joy and a sense of accomplishment, which can improve mood and reduce stress (Baker, Skolnik, Park, Sprich, & Wilhelm, 2023).

4. **Exposure Therapy:**

a. **Concept:** Exposure therapy involves gradually confronting feared situations or stimuli in a controlled and systematic manner to reduce avoidance behaviours and anxiety (Santos et al., 2023).

b. **Application:** By facing your fears in a safe environment, you learn that your anxiety decreases over time and that you can cope with the feared situation.

5. **Stress Inoculation Training (SIT)**

a. **Concept:** Stress Inoculation Training (SIT) is a CBT technique designed to help you develop coping skills to manage stress more effectively. You learn specific coping skills, such as relaxation techniques, cognitive restructuring, and problem-solving strategies which are then practiced in increasingly stressful situation to build resilience and confidence in managing stress (Knowles & Tolin, 2022).

b. **Application:** Techniques such as brainstorming, evaluating options, and implementing solutions are used to address specific problems and reduce stress.

Examples of CBT Techniques for Managing Stress

1. **Thought Records:**

a. **Description:** Thought records are worksheets used to identify and challenge negative automatic thoughts. You record the situation, your thoughts, emotions, and evidence for and against your thoughts.

b. **Example:** A person feeling anxious about a presentation might use a thought record to examine their fear of failure and identify more balanced thoughts, such as "I have prepared well and can handle this."

2. **Socratic Questioning:**

a. **Description:** Socratic questioning involves asking open-ended questions to help you critically examine your thoughts and beliefs.

b. **Example:** Questions like "What evidence do I have for this thought?" and "What is an alternative explanation?" can help challenge negative thinking patterns.

3. **Behavioural Experiments:**

a. **Description:** Behavioural experiments are planned activities designed to test the validity of negative beliefs and assumptions.

b. **Example:** Someone who believes they will be rejected if they ask for help might conduct an experiment by asking a colleague for assistance and observing the outcome.

4. **Activity Scheduling:**

a. **Description:** Activity scheduling involves planning and engaging in enjoyable and meaningful activities to improve mood and reduce stress.

b. **Example:** Scheduling regular exercise, hobbies, or social activities can provide a sense of accomplishment and enhance well-being.

Research Findings: Effectiveness of CBT in Reducing Stress-Related Disorders

1. **General Effectiveness Across Conditions:**

a. **Meta-Review and Panoramic Meta-Analysis:** A comprehensive meta-review published in *Psychological Medicine* summarized the evidence from 494 systematic reviews, representing over 221,000 participants. The study found that CBT produced a modest but consistent benefit across various conditions, including both mental and physical health issues (Fordham et al., 2021).

2. **Effectiveness for Anxiety Disorders:**

   a. **Systematic Review and Meta-Analysis:** A study published in *JAMA Psychiatry* assessed the long-term outcomes of CBT for anxiety disorders, PTSD, and OCD. The review included randomized controlled trials (RCTs) comparing CBT with care as usual, relaxation, psychoeducation, pill placebo, supportive therapy, or waiting list controls. The findings indicated that CBT had significant long-term benefits in reducing symptoms of anxiety, PTSD, and OCD (van Dis et al., 2020).

3. **Effectiveness for Stress-Related Disorders:**

   a. **Review in BioPsychoSocial Medicine:** A review published in *BioPsychoSocial Medicine* evaluated the effectiveness of CBT in managing stress-related disorders. The study found that CBT helps individuals eliminate avoidant and safety-seeking behaviours, facilitating stress management and reducing stress-related disorders (Nakao, Shirotsuki, & Sugaya, 2021). The review highlighted the importance of cognitive restructuring and behavioural activation in improving the ability to cope with stress.

Chapter 5

Building Resilience

We will now look at building resilience for stress management. Building resilience is essential because it equips you with the ability to adapt to and recover from stressful situations, thereby reducing the overall impact of stress on your life. By fostering resilience, you can maintain a positive outlook and effectively navigate challenges, which is crucial for long-term mental health and well-being. It is important to focus on building resilience as it not only helps in managing current stress but also prepares you to handle future adversities more effectively.

Incorporating Mindfulness into Daily Routines to Enhance Resilience for Stress Management

Mindfulness practices can be seamlessly integrated into daily routines to help manage stress and enhance resilience. These practices involve maintaining a present-centred awareness and a non-judgmental attitude towards thoughts and feelings. By incorporating these mindfulness practices into daily routines, you can effectively manage stress, enhance resilience, and improve your overall quality of life.

1. **Mindful Breathing:**
   a. **Concept:** Mindful breathing involves focusing on the breath and observing its natural rhythm without trying to change it. This practice helps anchor the mind in the present moment and reduce stress (Zeidan, Johnson, Gordon, & Goolkasian, 2010).
   b. **Technique:** Sit or lie down in a comfortable position. Close your eyes and take a few deep breaths. Focus on the sensation of your breath entering and leaving your body. If your mind wanders, gently bring your attention back to your breath.

2. **Body Scan Meditation:**
   a. **Concept:** Body scan meditation involves mentally scanning your body from head to toe, paying attention to any sensations, tension, or discomfort. This practice increases body awareness and promotes relaxation (Goyal et al., 2014).
   b. **Technique:** Lie down in a comfortable position. Close your eyes and take a few deep breaths. Slowly bring your attention to each part of your body, starting from your toes and moving up to your head. Notice any sensations without judgment.

3. **Mindful Eating:**
   a. **Concept:** Mindful eating involves paying full attention to the experience of eating, including the taste, texture, and smell of food. This practice helps cultivate a healthy relationship with food and reduces stress related to eating (Allen, Romate, & Rajkumar, 2021).
   b. **Technique:** Before eating, take a moment to appreciate the food. Eat slowly and savour each bite, paying attention to the flavours and textures. Avoid distractions such as TV or smartphones while eating.

4. **Mindful Walking:**
   a. **Concept:** Mindful walking involves walking slowly and deliberately, paying attention to the sensations of each step and the environment around you. This practice helps ground the mind and reduce stress (Burdick & Camhi, 2024).
   b. **Technique:** Find a quiet place to walk. Walk slowly and focus on the sensations of your feet touching the ground, the movement of your legs, and the rhythm of your breath. Notice the sights, sounds, and smells around you.

5. **Mindful Listening:**
   a. **Concept:** Mindful listening involves fully focusing on the sounds around you, whether it's music, nature

sounds, or a conversation. This practice helps improve concentration and reduce stress (Taraban, Heide, Woollacott, & Chan, 2017).

b. **Technique:** Sit or lie down in a comfortable position. Close your eyes and focus on the sounds around you. Notice the different layers of sound without judgment. If your mind wanders, gently bring your attention back to the sounds.

6. **Mindful Writing:**

a. **Concept:** Mindful writing is a practice that combines the principles of mindfulness with the act of writing. It involves being fully present and engaged in the writing process, paying attention to thoughts, feelings, and sensations without judgment. Colouring has also been found to significantly reduces stress and increases relaxation (Ashdown et al., 2018).

b. **Technique:** To practice mindful writing, find a quiet space, set an intention, and write freely without worrying about grammar or structure, focusing on the present moment and your thoughts. Periodically pause to reflect on what you've written and end by expressing gratitude for the insights gained.

1. **Morning Routine:**
   a. **Mindful Breathing:** Spend 5 minutes each morning sitting quietly and focusing on your breath before starting your daily activities.

2. **Work Breaks:**
   a. **Mindful Walking:** Spend 10 minutes walking mindfully around your office building or a nearby park during your lunch break.

3. **Meals:**
   a. **Mindful Eating:** Dedicate at least one meal each day to mindful eating, focusing on the taste, texture, and smell of your food.

4. **Evening Routine:**
   a. **Body Scan Meditation:** Spend 10-15 minutes each evening lying down and performing a body scan meditation before going to bed.

Benefits of Mindfulness: Improved Emotional Regulation and Stress Management

Improved Emotional Regulation

Mindfulness involves paying attention to the present moment with an attitude of openness and non-judgment. This practice can significantly improve emotional regulation by helping you become more aware of your emotions and respond to them in healthier ways.

1. **Awareness and Acceptance**: Mindfulness encourages awareness of one's emotional state without immediate reaction. This awareness allows you to recognize your emotions and understand your triggers. For example, if someone feels anger rising during a stressful situation, mindfulness helps them notice this emotion early and choose a more constructive response rather than reacting impulsively (Raugh, Berglund, & Strauss, 2024).

2. **Neuroscientific Evidence**: Research shows that mindfulness practices can lead to changes in brain regions associated with emotion regulation. For instance, increased activity in the prefrontal cortex (responsible for executive functions) and decreased activity in the amygdala (involved in emotional reactivity) have been observed in individuals who practice mindfulness regularly (Wheeler, Arnkoff, & Glass, 2017). This shift helps in better managing emotional responses.

3. **Practical Applications**: Mindfulness-Based Stress Reduction (MBSR) and Mindfulness-Based Cognitive Therapy (MBCT) are structured programs that incorporate mindfulness to help you manage emotions. These programs have been shown to reduce symptoms

of anxiety and depression by promoting healthier emotional processing (Guendelman, Medeiros, & Rampes, 2017).

Stress Management

By fostering a state of calm and focused awareness, mindfulness helps you cope with stress more effectively.

1. **Reduction in Stress Hormones:** Studies have found that mindfulness practices can reduce levels of cortisol. Lower cortisol levels are associated with reduced stress and improved overall health (Vargas-Uricoechea et al., 2024).

2. **Improved Coping Mechanisms:** Mindfulness teaches you to approach stressors with a non-judgmental attitude, which can prevent the escalation of stress. For example, during a high-pressure work situation, a mindful approach might involve taking a few deep breaths and observing one's thoughts and feelings without getting overwhelmed by them (Vargas-Uricoechea et al., 2024).

3. **Enhanced Resilience:** Regular mindfulness practice can build resilience, making you better equipped to handle future stressors. This resilience is partly due to the development of a more balanced perspective on

challenges and a greater sense of control over one's reactions (Vargas-Uricoechea et al., 2024).

Social Support: The Role of a Supportive Network in Managing Stress

Social support refers to the emotional, instrumental, and informational assistance provided by others. It can come from family, friends, colleagues, or community members and plays a significant role in managing stress.

1. **Emotional Support:** This involves expressions of empathy, love, trust, and caring. For example, having a friend who listens to your problems and offers comfort can help alleviate feelings of stress and anxiety.

2. **Instrumental Support:** This includes tangible aid and services that directly assist a person in need. For instance, a colleague helping you with a work task can reduce your workload and stress.

3. **Informational Support:** This involves providing advice, suggestions, and information that a person can use to address problems. For example, receiving guidance on how to handle a stressful situation can help you feel more equipped to manage it.

Benefits of Social Support

1. **Stress Buffering:** Social support acts as a buffer against stress. According to the buffering hypothesis, social support protects individuals from the harmful effects of stress by providing resources that help them cope more effectively (Acoba, 2024). For example, during a stressful life event like a job loss, having a supportive network can provide emotional comfort and practical assistance, reducing the overall impact of the stressor.

2. **Improved Mental Health:** Research has shown that social support is associated with lower levels of anxiety and depression. Research has found that perceived social support can mediate the relationship between stress and mental health outcomes, such as positive affect and reduced anxiety (Acoba, 2024). This means that individuals who feel supported are better able to manage stress and maintain better mental health.

3. **Enhanced Coping Mechanisms:** Social support can enhance an individual's coping mechanisms by providing different perspectives and solutions to problems. For example, discussing a stressful situation with friends can lead to new insights and coping strategies that you might not have considered on your own.

4. **Physiological Benefits:** Social support has been linked to lower levels of cortisol. Lower cortisol levels are associated with reduced stress and better overall health (Schmiedl, Schulte, & Kauffeld, 2022). Additionally, social interactions can trigger the release of oxytocin, a hormone that promotes feelings of bonding and reduces stress.

Creating a Supportive Environment: Tips for Fostering Supportive Relationships at Home and Work

Tips for fostering supportive relationships at home include:

1. **Open Communication:** Encourage open and honest communication within the family. This involves actively listening to each other without judgment and expressing thoughts and feelings openly. For example, regular family meetings can provide a platform for everyone to share their experiences and concerns.

2. **Show Appreciation:** Regularly express appreciation and gratitude for each other. Simple gestures like saying "thank you" or acknowledging someone's efforts can strengthen bonds. Expressing gratitude can enhance relationship satisfaction and reduce stress.

3. **Spend Quality Time Together:** Make time for family activities that everyone enjoys. This could be as simple as having dinner together, playing games, or going for a

walk. Quality time helps build strong emotional connections and provides opportunities for support during stressful times.

4. **Provide Emotional Support:** Be there for each other during tough times. Offering a listening ear, a comforting hug, or words of encouragement can make a significant difference. Emotional support helps you feel valued and understood, which can reduce stress.

5. **Create a Positive Environment:** Foster a positive and nurturing home environment. This includes maintaining a balance between work and family life, setting boundaries, and creating a space where everyone feels safe and respected.

Tips for fostering supportive relationships at work include:

1. **Encourage Team Collaboration:** Promote a culture of teamwork and collaboration. Encourage employees to work together on projects and support each other. Collaborative environments can reduce stress by sharing the workload and providing mutual support.

2. **Provide Constructive Feedback:** Offer constructive feedback and recognition for a job well done. Positive reinforcement can boost morale and create a supportive work atmosphere. Regular feedback helps employees feel valued and motivated.

3. **Promote Work-Life Balance:** Encourage employees to maintain a healthy work-life balance. This can include flexible working hours, remote work options, and promoting the importance of taking breaks. A balanced approach helps reduce stress and prevent burnout.

4. **Foster Open Communication:** Create an environment where employees feel comfortable sharing their concerns and ideas. Regular team meetings and one-on-one check-ins can facilitate open communication and provide opportunities for support.

5. **Offer Support Programs:** Implement support programs such as employee assistance programs (EAPs), mental health resources, and stress management workshops. These programs provide employees with the tools and resources they need to manage stress effectively.

Conclusion

Throughout this book, we have explored a variety of research supported methods for managing stress, each designed to help you lead a healthier and more balanced life. We began by defining stress and understanding its physiological and hormonal underpinnings, as well as the different types of stress and their impacts on health. From there, we delved into lifestyle modifications, highlighting the importance of quality sleep, regular exercise, a balanced diet, and effective time management in mitigating stress. We also examined various relaxation techniques, such as progressive muscle relaxation, diaphragmatic breathing, mindfulness meditation, aromatherapy, and hot and cold therapy, all of which can help activate the body's relaxation response and reduce stress levels.

In addition, we discussed the principles and effectiveness of cognitive-behavioural therapy (CBT) in managing stress by changing thought patterns and behaviours. We also emphasized the importance of building resilience through mindfulness practices and the support of a strong social network. While this book provides a thorough overview of these methods, it is not an exhaustive list. It is crucial to consult a medical professional before undertaking any new stress management techniques, especially if you are experiencing significant stress. A healthcare provider can offer personalized advice and ensure that the methods you choose are safe and appropriate for your specific circumstances. By understanding stress and employing research backed strategies, you can take control of your stress levels and improve your quality of life.

If you found this book resourceful, be sure to check out a free weekly newsletter at **www.ebsm.com.au** where we dive into different research studies that explore evidence-based stress management techniques. And check us out on Facebook and Instagram at **Evidence Based Stress Management.** Thank you for taking the time to read our book and we wish you all the best with taking control of the stress in your life.

Creating a personalized stress management plan is a proactive way to handle stress effectively. Here's a step-by-step guide to help you develop a plan tailored to your needs, incorporating techniques that work best for you:

Step 1: Identify Your Stressors

Start by identifying the sources of your stress. These can be external (e.g. work, relationships) or internal (e.g. self-criticism, unrealistic expectations). Keeping a stress journal can help you track situations that cause stress and your reactions to them, allowing you to identify patterns and specific triggers.

Step 2: Assess Your Current Coping Strategies

Evaluate how you currently cope with stress. Are these strategies effective, or do they contribute to more stress? Reflect on whether you tend to avoid stressors, confront them head-on, or use unhealthy coping mechanisms like overeating or excessive screen time.

Step 3: Trial Stress Management Techniques

As you explore the stress management techniques highlighted in this book, it's important to trial each method to see which ones work best for you. Some techniques may resonate more than others, and it's perfectly normal for certain methods to be more effective in conjunction with each other. For example, combining mindfulness meditation with regular physical activity might provide a more comprehensive stress relief than either technique alone. Additionally, it may take some time to notice changes in your stress levels, so be patient and give each method a fair trial. Remember, the goal is to find a personalized approach to stress management that fits your unique needs and lifestyle.

Step 4: Create Your Personalized Plan

Based on your assessment, create a plan that incorporates the techniques that work best for you. Be specific about how and when you will use these strategies.

- **Example:**
  - o **Morning Routine:** Start the day with 10 minutes of meditation.
  - o **Work Breaks:** Take short walks or practice deep breathing exercises.
  - o **Evening Routine:** Engage in a relaxing hobby like reading or listening to music.
  - o **Weekly Activities:** Schedule regular exercise and social activities with friends or family.

Step 5: Set Realistic Goals

Set achievable goals for incorporating these techniques into your daily life. Start small and gradually build up. For example, aim to meditate for 5 minutes each day for the first week, then gradually increase the duration.

Step 6: Monitor and Adjust

Regularly review your stress management plan and make adjustments as needed. Pay attention to what works and what doesn't, and be flexible in adapting your plan. For example, if you find that evening walks help you unwind better than reading, adjust your plan to include more walks.

Step 7: Seek Professional Help if Needed

If stress becomes overwhelming, consider seeking help from a therapist or counsellor. Professional guidance can provide additional support and effective coping strategies.

By taking these steps, you can develop a personalized stress management plan that helps you navigate life's challenges with greater ease and resilience. Remember, managing stress is a journey, and finding the right combination of techniques that work for you is key to achieving long-term well-being.

References

- Abdelhalim, A. R. (2021). The effect of Mentha piperita L. on the mental health issues of university students: A pilot study. *Journal of Pharmacy & Pharmacognosy Research, 9*(1), 49-57. https://doi.org/10.56499/jppres20.932_9.1.49

- Acoba, E. F. (2024). Social support and mental health: The mediating role of perceived stress. *Frontiers in Psychology, 15,* Article 1330720. https://doi.org/10.3389/fpsyg.2024.1330720

- Allen, J. G., Romate, J., & Rajkumar, E. (2021). Mindfulness-based positive psychology interventions: A systematic review. *BMC Psychology, 9,* Article 116. https://doi.org/10.1186/s40359-021-00618-2

- Anglin, R. E. S., Samaan, Z., Walter, S. D., & McDonald, S. D. (2013). Vitamin D deficiency and depression in adults: Systematic review and meta-analysis. *The British Journal of Psychiatry, 202*(2), 100-107. https://doi.org/10.1192/bjp.bp.111.106666

- Ashdown, B. K., Bodenlos, J. S., Arroyo, K., Patterson, M., Parkins, E., & Burstein, S. (2018). How does

coloring influence mood, stress, and mindfulness?
Journal of Integrated Social Sciences, *8*(1), 1-21.
https://www.jiss.org/documents/volume_8/JISS%20201
8%208%281%29%201-
21%20Coloring%20and%20Mindfulness.pdf

- Bahcecioglu Turan, G., Gürcan, F., & Özer, Z. (2023).
  The effects of eye masks and earplugs on sleep quality,
  anxiety, fear, and vital signs in patients in an intensive
  care unit: A randomised controlled study. *Journal of
  Sleep Research,* *32*(3), e14044.
  https://doi.org/10.1111/jsr.14044

- Baker, A. W., Skolnik, A. M., Park, J. M., Sprich, S. E.,
  & Wilhelm, S. (2023). Basic principles and practice of
  cognitive-behavioral therapy. In S. E. Sprich, & S.
  Wilhelm (Eds.), *The Massachusetts General Hospital
  Handbook of Cognitive Behavioral Therapy* (pp. 7-17).
  Springer. https://doi.org/10.1007/978-3-031-29368-9_2

- Bankenahally, R., & Krovvidi, H. (2016). Autonomic
  nervous system: Anatomy, physiology, and relevance in
  anaesthesia and critical care medicine. *BJA Education,*
  16(11), 381-387. https://doi.org/10.1093/bjaed/mkw011

- Bentley, T. G. K., D'Andrea-Penna, G., Rakic, M.,
  Arce, N., LaFaille, M., Berman, R., Cooley, K., &
  Sprimont, P. (2023). Breathing practices for stress and

anxiety reduction: Conceptual framework of implementation guidelines based on a systematic review of the published literature. *Brain Sciences, 13*(12), 1612. https://doi.org/10.3390/brainsci13121612

- Blaxton, J. M., Bergeman, C. S., Whitehead, B. R., Braun, M. E., & Payne, J. D. (2017). Relationships among nightly sleep quality, daily stress, and daily affect. *The Journals of Gerontology: Series B, 72*(3), 363-372. https://doi.org/10.1093/geronb/gbv060

- Bleakley, C. M., & Davison, G. W. (2010). What is the biochemical and physiological rationale for using cold-water immersion in sports recovery? A systematic review. *British Journal of Sports Medicine, 44*(3), 179-187. https://doi.org/10.1136/bjsm.2009.065565

- Blum, K. (2024). The impact of chronic stress on brain function and structure. *Neuroscience and Psychiatry: Open Access, 7*(5), 262-264. https://doi.org/10.47532/npoa.2024.7(5).262-264

- Burdick, A. V., & Camhi, S. M. (2024). The effects of a guided mindful walk on mental health in university students. *International Journal of Exercise Science, 17*(5), 590-601. https://digitalcommons.wku.edu/ijes/vol17/iss5/5/

- Byrnes, K., Wu, P.-J., & Whillier, S. (2017). Is Pilates an effective rehabilitation tool? A systematic review. *Journal of Bodywork and Movement Therapies, 21*(4), 752-762. https://doi.org/10.1016/j.jbmt.2017.04.005

- Caldwell, K., Harrison, M., Adams, M., & Triplett, N. T. (2009). Effect of Pilates and taiji quan training on self-efficacy, sleep quality, mood, and physical performance of college students. *Complementary Therapies in Clinical Practice, 15*(3), 141-146. https://doi.org/10.1016/j.ctcp.2009.06.002

- Chems-Maarif, R., Cavanagh, K., Baer, R., Gu, J., & Strauss, C. (2025). Defining mindfulness: A review of existing definitions and suggested refinements. *Mindfulness, 16*(1), 1-20. https://doi.org/10.1007/s12671-024-02507-2

- Chen, X., Touyz, R. M., Park, J. B., & Schiffrin, E. L. (2001). Antioxidant effects of vitamins C and E are associated with altered activation of vascular NADPH oxidase and superoxide dismutase in stroke-prone SHR. *Hypertension, 38*(2), 606-611. https://doi.org/10.1161/hy09t1.094005

- Czeisler, C. A., Buxton, O. M., & Dzierzewski, J. M. (2023). The importance of sleep regularity: A consensus statement of the National Sleep Foundation sleep timing and variability panel. *Sleep Health, 9*(6), 801-820. https://doi.org/10.1016/j.sleh.2023.07.016

- Datta, D., & Arnsten, A. F. T. (2019). Loss of prefrontal cortical higher cognition with uncontrollable stress: Molecular mechanisms, changes with age, and relevance to treatment. *Brain Sciences, 9*(5), 113. https://doi.org/10.3390/brainsci9050113

- Eberth, J., & Sedlmeier, P. (2012). The effects of mindfulness meditation: A meta-analysis. *Mindfulness, 3*(3), 174-189. https://doi.org/10.1007/s12671-012-0101-x

- Eissa, M. A., & Kader, F. A. A. (2015). Effectiveness of time management strategies instruction on students' academic time management and academic self-efficacy. *International Journal of Psycho-Educational Sciences, 4*(1), 45-52. https://files.eric.ed.gov/fulltext/ED565629.pdf

- Eldeeb, G. A. E., & Eldosoky, E. K. (2016). Relationship between effectiveness of time management and stress levels among nursing students. *IOSR Journal of Nursing and Health Science, 5*(2), 95-100. https://www.iosrjournals.org/iosr-jnhs/papers/vol5-issue2/Version-4/L05020495100.pdf

- Ernst, H., Scherpf, M., Pannasch, S., Helmert, J. R., Malberg, H., & Schmidt, M. (2023). Assessment of the human response to acute mental stress–An overview and a multimodal study. *PLOS ONE, 18*(11), e0294069.

- Fenn, K., & Byrne, M. (2013). The key principles of cognitive behavioural therapy. *InnovAiT, 6*(9), 579–585. https://doi.org/10.1177/1755738012471029

- Flinders University. (2024). Wake-up call for us all to establish regular healthy sleep patterns. *ScienceDaily.* Retrieved from https://www.sciencedaily.com/releases/2024/02/240222214147.htm

- Fordham, B., Sugavanam, T., Edwards, K., Stallard, P., Howard, R., das Nair, R., Copsey, B., Lee, H., Howick, J., & Hemming, K. (2021). The evidence for cognitive behavioural therapy in any condition, population or context: A meta-review of systematic reviews and panoramic meta-analysis. *Psychological Medicine, 51*(1), 21-29. https://doi.org/10.1017/S0033291720005292

- Gangadharan, P., & Madani, A. H. (2018). Effectiveness of progressive muscle relaxation techniques on depression, anxiety and stress among undergraduate nursing students. *International Journal of Health*

Sciences and Research, *8*(2), 147-154. https://www.ijhsr.org/IJHSR_Vol.8_Issue.2_Feb2018/2 0.pdf

- Garbarino, S., Lanteri, P., Bragazzi, N. L., Magnavita, N., & Scoditti, E. (2021). Role of sleep deprivation in immune-related disease risk and outcomes. *Communications Biology,* *4*, Article 2825. https://doi.org/10.1038/s42003-021-02825-4

- Goyal, M., Singh, S., Sibinga, E. M., Gould, N. F., Rowland-Seymour, A., Sharma, R., Berger, Z., Sleicher, D., Maron, D. D., Shihab, H. M., Ranasinghe, P. D., Linn, S., Saha, S., Bass, E. B., & Haythornthwaite, J. A. (2014). Meditation programs for psychological stress and well-being: A systematic review and meta-analysis. *JAMA Internal Medicine,* *174*(3), 357-368. https://doi.org/10.1001/jamainternmed.2013.13018

- Greco, V., Bergamo, D., Cuoccio, P., Konkoly, K. R., Lombardo, K. M., & Lewis, P. A. (2023). Wearing an eye mask during overnight sleep improves episodic learning and alertness. *Sleep,* *46*(3), zsac305. https://doi.org/10.1093/sleep/zsac305

- Guendelman, S., Medeiros, S., & Rampes, H. (2017). Mindfulness and emotion regulation: Insights from neurobiological, psychological, and clinical studies.

Frontiers in Psychology, 8, Article 220. https://doi.org/10.3389/fpsyg.2017.00220

- Halbreich, U. (2021). Stress-related physical and mental disorders: A new paradigm. *BJPsych Advances, 27*(3), 145-152. https://doi.org/10.1192/bja.2021.1

- Halkos, G., & Bousinakis, D. (2010). The effect of stress and satisfaction on productivity. *International Journal of Productivity and Performance Management, 59*(5), 415-431. https://doi.org/10.1108/17410401011052869

- Hamasaki, H. (2020). Effects of diaphragmatic breathing on health: A narrative review. *Medicines, 7*(10), 65. https://doi.org/10.3390/medicines7100065

- Hamblin, M. R. (2017). Mechanisms and applications of the anti-inflammatory effects of photobiomodulation. *AIMS Biophysics, 4*(3), 337-361. https://doi.org/10.3934/biophy.2017.3.337

- Heijnen, S., Hommel, B., Kibele, A., & Colzato, L. S. (2016). Neuromodulation of aerobic exercise—A review. *Frontiers in Psychology, 6,* 1890. https://doi.org/10.3389/fpsyg.2015.01890

- Herz, R. S. (2009). Aromatherapy facts and fictions: A scientific analysis of olfactory effects on mood, physiology and behavior. *International Journal of*

Neuroscience, 119(2), 263-290. https://doi.org/10.1080/00207450802333953

- Hofmann, S. G., & Gómez, A. F. (2017). Mindfulness-based interventions for anxiety and depression. *Psychiatric Clinics of North America, 40*(4), 739-749. https://doi.org/10.1016/j.psc.2017.08.008

- Hofmann, S. G., & Gómez, A. F. (2017). Mindfulness-based interventions for anxiety and depression. *Psychiatric Clinics of North America, 40*(4), 739-749. https://doi.org/10.1016/j.psc.2017.08.008

- Hohenauer, E., Taeymans, J., Baeyens, J. P., Clarys, P., & Clijsen, R. (2015). The effect of post-exercise cryotherapy on recovery characteristics: A systematic review and meta-analysis. *PLoS ONE, 10*(9), e0139028. https://doi.org/10.1371/journal.pone.0139028

- Horovitz, O. (2025). Nutritional psychology: Review the interplay between nutrition and mental health. *Nutrition Reviews, 83*(3), 562-576. https://doi.org/10.1093/nutrit/nuae158

- Huhtaniemi, I. T., & Laukkanen, J. A. (2020). Endocrine effects of sauna bath. *Current Opinion in Endocrine and Metabolic Research, 11*, 15-20. https://doi.org/10.1016/j.coemr.2019.12.004

- Hussain, J., & Cohen, M. (2018). A hot topic for health: Results of the Global Sauna Survey. *Complementary Therapies in Medicine, 41*, 247-254. https://doi.org/10.1016/j.ctim.2018.10.013

- Huttunen, P., Kokko, L., & Ylijukuri, V. (2004). Winter swimming improves general well-being. *International Journal of Circumpolar Health, 63*(2), 140-144. https://doi.org/10.3402/ijch.v63i2.17700

- Ideaure. (2021). Spinner rings as stress relief: What science says about this trending anxiety aid. Retrieved from http://ideaure.com/blogs/news/spinner-rings-as-stress-relief-what-science-says-about-this-trending-anxiety-aid

- James, K. A., Stromin, J. I., Steenkamp, N., & Combrinck, M. I. (2023). Understanding the relationships between physiological and psychosocial stress, cortisol and cognition. *Frontiers in Endocrinology, 14*. Retrieved from Frontiers

- Jerath, R., Crawford, M. W., Barnes, V. A., & Harden, K. (2015). Self-regulation of breathing as a primary treatment for anxiety. *Applied Psychophysiology and Biofeedback, 40*(2), 107-115. https://doi.org/10.1007/s10484-015-9279-8

- Kandel, E. R., Schwartz, J. H., Jessell, T. M., Siegelbaum, S. A., & Hudspeth, A. J. (2013). *Principles of Neural Science* (5th ed.). McGraw-Hill Education. Retrieved from Archive.org

- Khan, S., & Khan, R. A. (2017). Chronic stress leads to anxiety and depression. *Annals of Psychiatry and Mental Health,* *5*(1), 1091. Retrieved from https://www.jscimedcentral.com/public/assets/articles/p sychiatry-5-1091.pdf

- Khan, S., & Khan, R. A. (2017). Chronic stress leads to anxiety and depression. *Annals of Psychiatry and Mental Health,* *5*(1), 1091. Retrieved from https://www.jscimedcentral.com/public/assets/articles/p sychiatry-5-1091.pdf

- Khan, S., & Khan, R. A. (2017). Chronic stress leads to anxiety and depression. *Annals of Psychiatry and Mental Health,* *5*(1), 1091. Retrieved from https://www.jscimedcentral.com/public/assets/articles/p sychiatry-5-1091.pdf

- Kim, C. E., Shin, S., Lee, H. W., Lim, J., Lee, J. K., Shin, A., & Kang, D. (2018). Association between sleep duration and metabolic syndrome: A cross-sectional study. *BMC Public Health, 18,* Article 720. https://doi.org/10.1186/s12889-018-5557-8

- Knezevic, E., Nenic, K., Milanovic, V., & Knezevic, N. N. (2023). The role of cortisol in chronic stress, neurodegenerative diseases, and psychological disorders. *Cells, 12*(23), 2726. https://doi.org/10.3390/cells12232726

- Knowles, K. A., & Tolin, D. F. (2022). Mechanisms of action in exposure therapy. *Current Psychiatry Reports, 24*(11), 861–869. https://doi.org/10.1007/s11920-022-01391-8

- Koiler, R., Schimmel, A., Bakhshipour, E., Shewokis, P. A., & Getchell, N. (2022). The impact of fidget spinners on fine motor skills in individuals with and without ADHD: An exploratory analysis. *Journal of Behavioral and Brain Science, 12*(3), 82-101. https://doi.org/10.4236/jbbs.2022.123005

- Kopplin, C. S., & Rosenthal, L. (2022). The positive effects of combined breathing techniques and cold exposure on perceived stress: A randomised trial. *Current Psychology, 42,* 27058–27070. https://doi.org/10.1007/s12144-022-03739-y

- Korkutata, A., Korkutata, M., & Lazarus, M. (2024). The impact of exercise on sleep and sleep disorders. *Nature Mental Health, 1*(1), 18. https://doi.org/10.1038/s44323-024-00018-w

- Kris-Etherton, P. M., Petersen, K. S., Hibbeln, J. R., Hurley, D., Kolick, V., Peoples, S., Rodriguez, N., & Woodward-Lopez, G. (2021). Nutrition and behavioral health disorders: Depression and anxiety. *Nutrition Reviews, 79*(3), 247-260. https://doi.org/10.1093/nutrit/nuaa025

- Krugers, H. J., Lucassen, P. J., Karst, H., & Joëls, M. (2010). Chronic stress effects on hippocampal structure and synaptic function: Relevance for depression and normalization by anti-glucocorticoid treatment. *Frontiers in Synaptic Neuroscience, 2*, Article 24. https://doi.org/10.3389/fnsyn.2010.00024

- Kumutha, V., Aruna, S., & Poongodi, R. (2014). Effectiveness of progressive muscle relaxation technique on stress and blood pressure among elderly with hypertension. *IOSR Journal of Nursing and Health Science, 3*(4), 1-6. https://www.iosrjournals.org/iosr-jnhs/papers/vol3-issue4/Version-2/A03420106.pdf

- Law, R., & Clow, A. (2020). Stress, the cortisol awakening response and cognitive function. In A. Clow & N. Smyth (Eds.), *Stress and brain health: Across the life course* (pp. 187-217). Elsevier Academic Press. Retrieved from PsycNet

- Lee, J. H., Meyer, E. J., Nenke, M. A., Lightman, S. L., & Torpy, D. J. (2024). Cortisol, stress, and disease—Bidirectional associations; role for corticosteroid-binding globulin? *The Journal of Clinical Endocrinology & Metabolism, 109*(9), 2161-2172. Retrieved from Oxford Academic

- Lei, A. A., Phang, V. W. X., Lee, Y. Z., Kow, A. S. F., Tham, C. L., Ho, Y. C., & Lee, M. T. (2025). Chronic stress-associated depressive disorders: The impact of HPA axis dysregulation and neuroinflammation on the hippocampus—A mini review. *International Journal of Molecular Sciences, 26*(7), 2940. https://doi.org/10.3390/ijms26072940

- Liu, P. Z., & Nusslock, R. (2018). Exercise-mediated neurogenesis in the hippocampus via BDNF. *Frontiers in Neuroscience, 12,* 52. https://doi.org/10.3389/fnins.2018.00052

- Lo Martire, V., Berteotti, C., Zoccoli, G., & Bastianini, S. (2024). Improving sleep to improve stress resilience. *Current Sleep Medicine Reports, 10*(1), 23-33. https://doi.org/10.1007/s40675-024-00274-z

- Mah, L., Claudia, C., & Alexandra, H. (2016). Can anxiety damage the brain? *Current Opinion in Psychiatry, 29*(1), 10-15. Retrieved April 15, 2025, from https://journals.lww.com/co-psychiatry/abstract/2016/01000/can_anxiety_damage_the_brain_.10.aspx

- Manosso, L. M., Gasparini, C. R., Réus, G. Z., & Pavlovic, Z. M. (2022). Definitions and concepts of stress. In *Glutamate and Neuropsychiatric Disorders* (pp. 27-63). Springer. Retrieved from SpringerLink

- Marks, T. (2020). Creating restful environments: Applying evidenced-based interventions to increase the patients' perceptions of room quietness at night. Retrieved from https://www.academia.edu/79159164/Creating_Restful_Environments_Applying_Evidenced_Based_Interventi ons_to_Increase_the_Patients_Perceptions_of_Room_Quietness_at_Night

- Marques, A., Marconcin, P., Werneck, A. O., Ferrari, G., Gouveia, É. R., Kliegel, M., Peralta, M., & Ihle, A. (2021). Bidirectional association between physical activity and dopamine across adulthood—A systematic review. *Brain Sciences, 11*(7), 829. https://doi.org/10.3390/brainsci11070829

- Miao, X. R., Chen, Q. B., Wei, K., Tao, K. M., & Lu, Z. J. (2018). Posttraumatic stress disorder: From diagnosis to prevention. *Military Medical Research, 5*(1), 32. https://doi.org/10.1186/s40779-018-0179-0

- Nakao, M., Shirotsuki, K., & Sugaya, N. (2021). Cognitive–behavioral therapy for management of mental health and stress-related disorders: Recent advances in techniques and technologies. *BioPsychoSocial Medicine, 15*, Article 16. https://doi.org/10.1186/s13030-021-00219-w

103

- Nakao, M., Shirotsuki, K., & Sugaya, N. (2021). Cognitive-behavioral therapy for management of mental health and stress-related disorders: Recent advances in techniques and technologies. *BioPsychoSocial Medicine, 15*, Article 16. https://doi.org/10.1186/s13030-021-00219-w

- Nater, U. M. (2021). Recent developments in stress and anxiety research. *Journal of Neural Transmission, 128*(9), 1265-1267. Retrieved from SpringerLink

- Owen, L., & Corfe, B. (2017). The role of diet and nutrition on mental health and wellbeing. *Proceedings of the Nutrition Society, 76*(4), 425-426. https://doi.org/10.1017/S0029665117001057

- Pahomov, N. V., Kostunina, D. S., & Artemenkov, A. A. (2024). The influence of physical activity on the level of chronic inflammation in health and in noninfectious diseases. *Human Physiology, 50*(3), 293-299. https://doi.org/10.1134/S0362119723600595

- Pan, R., Zhang, G., Deng, F., Lin, W., & Pan, J. (2023). Effects of red light on sleep and mood in healthy subjects and individuals with insomnia disorder. *Frontiers in Psychiatry, 14*, Article 1200350. https://doi.org/10.3389/fpsyt.2023.1200350

- Pascoe, M. C., Thompson, D. R., Jenkins, Z. M., & Ski, C. F. (2017). Yoga, mindfulness-based stress reduction and stress-related physiological measures: A meta-analysis. *Psychoneuroendocrinology, 86,* 152-168. https://doi.org/10.1016/j.psyneuen.2017.08.008

- Paula, D., Luís, P., Pereira, O. R., & João, S. M. (2017). Aromatherapy in the control of stress and anxiety. *Alternative and Integrative Medicine, 6*(4). https://doi.org/10.4172/2327-5162.1000248

- Perciavalle, V., Blandini, M., Fecarotta, P., Buscemi, A., Di Corrado, D., Bertolo, L., Fichera, F., & Coco, M. (2017). The role of deep breathing on stress. *Neurological Sciences, 38*(3), 451-458. https://doi.org/10.1007/s10072-016-2790-8

- Persia, J. (2023). Examining the impacts of subtle fidget jewelry on anxiety, stress, and attention. *Carolina Digital Repository.* https://cdr.lib.unc.edu/concern/honors_theses/n87102 128

- Pinckard, K., Baskin, K. K., & Stanford, K. I. (2019). Effects of exercise to improve cardiovascular health. *Frontiers in Cardiovascular Medicine, 6,* 69. https://doi.org/10.3389/fcvm.2019.00069

- Prochilo, G. A., Costa, R. J. S., Hassed, C., Chambers, R., & Molenberghs, P. (2021). A 16-week aerobic exercise and mindfulness-based intervention on chronic psychosocial stress: A pilot and feasibility study. *Pilot and Feasibility Studies, 7,* 64. https://doi.org/10.1186/s40814-020-00751-6

- Raugh, I. M., Berglund, A. M., & Strauss, G. P. (2024). Implementation of mindfulness-based emotion regulation strategies: A systematic review and meta-analysis. *Affective Science, 6*(1), 171–200. https://doi.org/10.1007/s42761-024-00281-x

- Regenus Center. (2024). Can red light therapy improve mood? Retrieved from https://regenuscenter.com/red-light-therapy-faq/can-red-light-therapy-improve-mood/

- Reilly, E. B., & Stuyvenberg, C. L. (2023). A meta-analysis of loving-kindness meditations on self-compassion. *Mindfulness, 14*(10), 2299-2310. https://doi.org/10.1007/s12671-022-01972-x

- Romeo, J., Wärnberg, J., Pozo, T., & Marcos, A. (2010). Physical activity, immunity and infection. *Proceedings of the Nutrition Society, 69*(3), 390-399. https://doi.org/10.1017/S0029665110001795

- Saiyudthong, S., Chansiri, K., Lee, B., Sittiprapaporn, P., & Sathirachawan, K. (2025). Acute and chronic effect of essential oil blend on physiological response of stress. *International Journal of Neuropsychopharmacology, 28*(Supplement_1), i369–i370. https://doi.org/10.1093/ijnp/pyae059.656

- Santos, B., Silva, C., Garrido, C., Pires, R., Monteso-Curto, P., & Sequeira, C. (2023). Efficacy of cognitive restructuring in people with depressive symptoms: A scoping review protocol. In E. Moguel et al. (Eds.), *Gerontechnology V* (pp. 251–259). Springer. https://doi.org/10.1007/978-3-031-29067-1_25

- Sapolsky, R. M., Romero, L. M., & Munck, A. U. (2000). How do glucocorticoids influence stress responses? Integrating permissive, suppressive, stimulatory, and preparative actions. *Endocrine Reviews, 21*(1), 55-89. https://doi.org/10.1210/edrv.21.1.0389

- Schenkel, E. J., Ciesla, R., & Shanga, G. M. (2018). Effects of nasal dilator strips on subjective measures of sleep in subjects with chronic nocturnal nasal congestion: A randomized, placebo-controlled trial. *Allergy, Asthma & Clinical Immunology, 14*, 34. https://doi.org/10.1186/s13223-018-0258-5

- Schmiedl, A., Schulte, E.-M., & Kauffeld, S. (2022). The demands-buffering role of perceived and received social support for perceived stress and cortisol levels. *European Journal of Health Psychology, 29*(4), 175-186. https://doi.org/10.1027/2512-8442/a000110

- Shahsavarani, A. M., Marz Abadi, E. A., & Kalkhoran, M. H. (2015). Stress: Facts and theories through literature review. *International Journal of Medical Reviews, 2*(2), 230-241. Retrieved from https://www.ijmedrev.com/article_68654_37adc02e943 2adfa017b8d6095cb6760.pdf

- Sharifi-Rad, M., Kumar, N. V. A., Zucca, P., Varoni, E. M., Dini, L., Panzarini, E., Rajkovic, J., Tsouh Fokou, P. V., Azzini, E., Peluso, I., Mishra, A. P., Nigam, M., El Rayess, Y., El Beyrouthy, M., Polito, L., Iriti, M., Martins, N., Martorell, M., Docea, A. O., Setzer, W. N., Calina, D., Cho, W. C., & Sharifi-Rad, J. (2020). Lifestyle, oxidative stress, and antioxidants: Back and forth in the pathophysiology of chronic diseases. *Frontiers in Physiology, 11*, 694. https://doi.org/10.3389/fphys.2020.00694

- Sharma, I. (2024). The role of neurotransmitters in emotional regulation. *International Journal of Indian Psychology, 12*(1), 114. https://doi.org/10.25215/1201.114

- Shchaslyvyi, A. Y., Antonenko, S. V., & Telegeev, G. D. (2024). Comprehensive review of chronic stress pathways and the efficacy of behavioral stress reduction programs (BSRPs) in managing diseases. *International Journal of Environmental Research and Public Health, 21*(8), 1077. https://doi.org/10.3390/ijerph21081077

- Sherman, B. E., Huang, I., Wijaya, E. G., Turk-Browne, N. B., & Goldfarb, E. V. (2024). Acute stress effects on statistical learning and episodic memory. *Journal of Cognitive Neuroscience, 36*(8), 1741-1759. https://doi.org/10.1162/jocn_a_02178

- Singh, B., Bennett, H., Miatke, A., Dumuid, D., Curtis, R., Ferguson, T., Brinsley, J., Szeto, K., Petersen, J. M., Gough, C., Eglitis, E., Simpson, C. E. M., Ekegren, C. L., Smith, A. E., Erickson, K. I., & Maher, C. (2025). Effectiveness of exercise for improving cognition, memory and executive function: A systematic umbrella review and meta-meta-analysis. *British Journal of Sports Medicine.* Advance online publication. https://doi.org/10.1136/bjsports-2024-108589

- Singh, B., Olds, T., Curtis, R., Dumuid, D., Virgara, R., Watson, A., Szeto, K., O'Connor, E., Ferguson, T., Eglitis, E., Miatke, A., Simpson, C. E. M., & Maher, C. (2023). Effectiveness of physical activity interventions for improving depression, anxiety and distress: An overview of systematic reviews. *British Journal of Sports Medicine, 57*(18), 1203-1209. https://doi.org/10.1136/bjsports-2022-106195

- Singh, L. K. (2017). Time management and its effect on stress level. *International Journal of Current Advanced Research,* *6*(12), 8336-8337. https://www.academia.edu/41429911/TIME_MANAG EMENT_AND_ITS_EFFECT_ON_STRESS_LEVE L

- Takagi, C., Nakagawa, S., Hirata, N., Ohta, S., & Shimoeda, S. (2019). Evaluating the effect of aromatherapy on a stress marker in healthy subjects. *Journal of Pharmaceutical Health Care and Sciences, 5,* Article 18. https://doi.org/10.1186/s40780-019-0148-0

- Taraban, O., Heide, F. J., Woollacott, M. H., & Chan, D. (2017). The effects of a mindful listening task on mind-wandering. *Mindfulness,* *8*(2), 433–443. https://doi.org/10.1007/s12671-016-0615-8

- Torres, R., Koutakis, P., & Forsse, J. S. (2021). The effects of different exercise intensities and modalities on cortisol production in healthy individuals: A review. *Journal of Exercise and Nutrition, 4*(4), 19. Retrieved from https://www.journalofexerciseandnutrition.com/index.p hp/JEN/article/view/108

- Tsakona, P., Kitsatis, I., Apostolou, T., Papadopoulou, O., & Hristara-Papadopoulou, A. (2025). The effect of diaphragmatic breathing as a complementary therapeutic strategy in stress of children and teenagers 6–18 years old. *Children, 12*(1), 59. https://doi.org/10.3390/children12010059

- Ullian, M. E. (1999). The role of corticosteroids in the regulation of vascular tone. *Cardiovascular Research, 41*(1), 55-64. Retrieved from Oxford Academic

- van Dis, E. A. M., van Veen, S. C., Hagenaars, M. A., Batelaan, N. M., Bockting, C. L. H., van den Heuvel, R. M., Cuijpers, P., & Engelhard, I. M. (2020). Long-term outcomes of cognitive behavioral therapy for anxiety-related disorders: A systematic review and meta-analysis. *JAMA Psychiatry, 77*(3), 265–273. https://doi.org/10.1001/jamapsychiatry.2019.3986

- Vargas-Uricoechea, H., Castellanos-Pinedo, A., Urrego-Noguera, K., Vargas-Sierra, H. D., Pinzón-Fernández, M. V., Barceló-Martínez, E., & Ramírez-Giraldo, A. F. (2024). Mindfulness-based interventions and the hypothalamic–pituitary–adrenal axis: A systematic review. *Neurology International, 16*(6), 1552-1584. https://doi.org/10.3390/neurolint16060115

- Watson, N. F., Badr, M. S., Belenky, G., Bliwise, D. L., Buxton, O. M., Buysse, D., Dinges, D. F., Gangwisch, J., Grandner, M. A., Kushida, C., Malhotra, R. K.,

Martin, J. L., Patel, S. R., Quan, S. F., & Tasali, E. (2015). Recommended amount of sleep for a healthy adult: A joint consensus statement of the American Academy of Sleep Medicine and Sleep Research Society. *Journal of Clinical Sleep Medicine, 11*(6), 591-592. https://doi.org/10.5664/jcsm.4758

- Weber, J., Angerer, P., & Apolinário-Hagen, J. (2022). Physiological reactions to acute stressors and subjective stress during daily life: A systematic review on ecological momentary assessment (EMA) studies. *PLOS ONE, 17*(7), Article e0271996. https://doi.org/10.1371/journal.pone.0271996

- Wheeler, M. S., Arnkoff, D. B., & Glass, C. R. (2017). The neuroscience of mindfulness: How mindfulness alters the brain and facilitates emotion regulation. *Mindfulness, 8*(6), 1471–1487. https://doi.org/10.1007/s12671-017-0742-x

- Woo, H., Hong, C. J., Jung, S., Choe, S., & Yu, S. W. (2018). Chronic restraint stress induces hippocampal memory deficits by impairing insulin signalling. *Molecular Brain, 11*(37). https://doi.org/10.1186/s13041-018-0381-8

- Yu, W., Xiao, Y., Jayaraman, A., Yen, Y.-C., Lee, H. U., Pettersson, S., & Je, H. S. (2020). Microbial metabolites tune amygdala neuronal hyperexcitability and anxiety-linked behaviors. *Frontiers in Physiology, 11*, 694. https://doi.org/10.3389/fphys.2020.00694

- Zeidan, F., Johnson, S. K., Gordon, N. S., & Goolkasian, P. (2010). Effects of brief and sham mindfulness meditation on mood and cardiovascular variables. *Journal of Alternative and Complementary Medicine, 16*(8), 867-873. https://doi.org/10.1089/acm.2009.0321

- Zhang, X., Ge, T., Yin, G., Cui, R., Zhao, G., & Yang, W. (2018). Stress-induced functional alterations in amygdala: Implications for neuropsychiatric diseases. *Frontiers in Neuroscience, 12*(367). https://doi.org/10.3389/fnins.2018.00367

www.ingramcontent.com/pod-product-compliance
Lightning Source LLC
Chambersburg PA
CBHW070047100426
42740CB00013B/2832